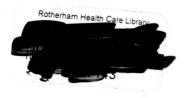

Acute Care

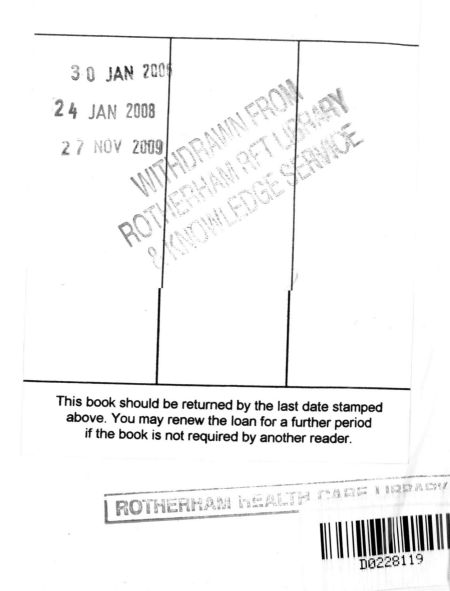

Acute Care Nurse Practitioner SECRETS

BARBARA A. TODD, MSN, CRNP, APRN-BC
Adjunct faculty
University of Pennsylvania;
Director, Clinical Surgical Specialists and Practitioners
Department of Surgery
The Hospital of the University of Pennsylvania
Philadelphia, Pennsylvania

SERIES EDITOR
LINDA SCHEETZ, EdD, APRN, BC, CEN
Assistant Professor
College of Nursing
Rutgers, The State University of New Jersey
Rutgers, New Jersey

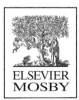

ELSEVIER
MOSBY

ELSEVIER
MOSBY

11830 Westline Industrial Drive
St. Louis, Missouri 63146

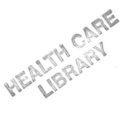

ACUTE CARE NURSE PRACTITIONER SECRETS   ISBN 0-323-03266-4
Copyright © 2005, Elsevier Inc.

NOTICE

International Standard Book Number 0-323-03266-4

Executive Publisher: Barbara Nelson Cullen
Editor: Sandra Clark Brown
Developmental Editor: Sophia Oh Gray
Publishing Services Manager: Deborah L. Vogel
Senior Project Manager: Jodi M. Willard
Design Project Manager: Bill Drone

Working together to grow
libraries in developing countries

www.elsevier.com | www.bookaid.org | www.sabre.org

ELSEVIER   BOOK AID International   Sabre Foundation

Printed in United States of America

Last digit is the print number: 9   8   7   6   5   4   3   2   1

I would like to dedicate this book to all my family, colleagues, and patients, who have taught me many lessons.

Contributors

KAREN CAMPBELL BETTEN, MSN, APRN, BC
Former Nurse Practitioner, Colon and Rectal Surgery
New York Presbyterian Hospital
Columbia University Medical Center
New York, New York
    8. Gastrointestinal Disorders

VIRGINIA BUCKLEY-BLASKOVICH, BSN, MSN, CRNP
Aortic Surgery Program Coordinator
Cardiothoracic Nurse Practitioner
The Hospital of the University of Pennsylvania
Philadelphia, Pennsylvania
    7. Cardiac Disorders

KATHRYN L. BURG, MSN, CRNP
Bariatric Surgery Program Coordinator
The Hospital of the University of Pennsylvania
Philadelphia, Pennsylvania
    8. Gastrointestinal Disorders

MEGAN E. CARR, MSN, CRNP, ACNP, BC, CCRN
Clinical Faculty
University of Pennsylvania
Philadelphia, Pennsylvania;
Nurse Practitioner, Medical ICU
The Hospital of the University of Pennsylvania
Philadelphia, Pennsylvania
    22. End-of-Life Issues

CATHERINE CRISTOFALO, MSN, CRNP, APRN-BC
Vascular Surgery Nurse Practitioner
The Hospital of the University of Pennsylvania
Philadelphia, Pennsylvania
    20. Pain Management

Sandra Davis, MSN, CRNP
Assistant Professor
Drexel University
Philadelphia, Pennsylvania;
Nurse Practitioner, Cardiothoracic Surgery
Abington Hospital
Abington, Pennsylvania
>   1. Common Laboratory Tests
>   5. Endocrine Disorders

Nancy Evans-Stoner, MSN, RN
Clinical Nurse Specialist, Clinical Nutrition Support Services
The Hospital of the University of Pennsylvania
Philadelphia, Pennsylvania
>   14. Nutrition Support

Colleen M. Harker, MSN, CRNP
Adjunct Faculty
The College of New Jersey
Ewing, New Jersey;
Surgical Oncology Nurse Practitioner
University of Pennsylvania Health System
Philadelphia, Pennsylvania
>   12. Hematological and Oncological Disorders

Rosanne Iacono, RNC, MSN, CRNP
Adjunct Faculty
University of Pennsylvania
Philadelphia, Pennsylvania;
Nurse Practitioner
Project Manager, Breast Cancer Prevention Program
Thomas Jefferson University
Philadelphia, Pennsylvania
>   13. Health Promotion

Eunice N. Jeon, MS, PA-C
Physician Assistant, Division of Urology
The Hospital of the University of Pennsylvania
Philadelphia, Pennsylvania
>   10. Renal and Genitourinary Disorders

Ruth M. Kleinpell, PhD, RN, FAAN, ACNP
Associate Professor
Rush University, College of Nursing
Chicago, Illinois; Nurse Practitioner
Our Lady of the Resurrection Medical Center
Chicago, Illinois
>   16. Sepsis and Septic Shock
>   18. Classifications of Shock

ANNE MARIE KUZMA, RN, MSN, CTTC
Lead Lung Transplant/Pulmonary Nurse Coordinator
Temple University Hospital
Philadelphia, Pennsylvania
  6. Pulmonary Disorders

JEAN DOUGHERTY LUCIANO, MSN, RN, CNRN, CRNP
Stroke Team Nurse Practitioner
The Hospital of the University of Pennsylvania
Philadelphia, Pennsylvania
  9. Neurological Disorders

MARY MacCORMACK-SUTER, MSN, CRNP
Clinical Director Cardiac and Thoracic Services
Temple University Hospital
Philadelphia, Pennsylvania
  3. Cardiac Diagnostic Studies

JAMES D. MENDEZ, MSN, CRNP
Nurse Practitioner
Program for Advanced Lung Disease and Lung Transplantation
The Hospital of the University of Pennsylvania
Philadelphia, Pennsylvania
  4. Pulmonary Diagnostic Studies

DENISE M. MEREDITH, RN, MSN, CRNP
Clinical Preceptor, Acute Care Nurse Practitioner Program
Surgical Critical Care Nurse Practitioner
Division of Traumatology and Surgical Critical Care
The Hospital of the University of Pennsylvania
Philadelphia, Pennsylvania
  19. Sedation Management

ANNEMARIE MURPHY, MSN, CRNP
Nurse Practitioner, Division of Vascular Surgery
The Hospital of the University of Pennsylvania
Philadelphia, Pennsylvania
  11. Musculoskeletal and Vascular Disorders

MARY LOU O'HARA, MSN, RN, CCRN
Clinical Research and Mechanical Assist Device Coordinator
The Hospital of the University of Pennsylvania
Philadelphia, Pennsylvania
  17. Advanced Cardiac Support Devices

PHYLLIS ANN SCHIAVONE-GATTO
Advanced Practice Nurse, Clinical Nutrition Support Services
The Hospital of the University of Pennsylvania
Philadelphia, Pennsylvania
  14. Nutrition Support

KATHLEEN SHAUGHNESSY, RN, MSN, CRNP
Nurse Practitioner, Clinical Instructor/Preceptor
Thomas Jefferson University
Philadelphia, Pennsylvania;
Nurse Practitioner, Cardiac Surgery
Abington Memorial Hospital
Abington, Pennsylvania
  2. Radiological Diagnostic Studies

CORINNA P. SICOUTRIS, MSN, CRNP, BC, CCRN
Surgical Critical Care Nurse Practitioner
The Hospital of the University of Pennsylvania
Philadelphia, Pennsylvania
  15. Traumatic Injuries

KAREN R. STEINKE, RN, MSN, CCTC
Transplant Coordinator
Temple University Hospital
Philadelphia, Pennsylvania
  6. Pulmonary Disorders

WENDY STEVENS, BSN, MSN, CRNP-BC, CCRN
Surgical Critical Care Nurse Practitioner
The Hospital of the University of Pennsylvania
Philadelphia, Pennsylvania
  21. Ventilator Management

CAROL TWOMEY, MSN, CRNP
Nurse Practitioner, Cardiac Surgery
The Hospital of the University of Pennsylvania
Philadelphia, Pennsylvania
  7. Cardiac Disorders

ANGELA M. VOTODIAN, MSN, CRNP
Acute Care Nurse Practitioner
The Hospital of the University of Pennsylvania
Philadelphia, Pennsylvania
  9. Neurological Disorders

Reviewers

Susan J. Appel, PhD, ACNP, FNP, BC, CCRN
Assistant Professor of Nursing
University of Alabama at Birmingham
Birmingham, Alabama

Lisa Latendresse, MBA, MSN, CCRN
LTC, United States Army
Graduate School of Nursing
Uniformed Services University
Bethesda, Maryland

Kara Laze, RN, MS, ACNP
Critical Care Nurse Practitioner
Pulmonary Medicine
University of Massachusetts Memorial Medical Center
Worcester, Massachusetts

Allyson Mobley, RN, BSN
Charge Nurse
Heart and Lung Transplant Intensive Care
University of Alabama at Birmingham
Birmingham, Alabama

Preface

The role of the acute care nurse practitioner (ACNP) continues to evolve. The expansion of the roles in the acute care setting has greatly increased the opportunities for the ACNP. *Acute Care Nurse Practitioner Secrets* is not meant to be a textbook but rather a series of key questions that you may confront as an ACNP. We teach by asking questions. I believe the best way to teach is to question. The authors of the chapters in this text represent NPs involved in various subspecialty practices in acute care.

The book is divided into three sections. Section I is dedicated to diagnostic studies and their clinical implications. Section II focuses on common issues in acute care. Each chapter in this section discusses medical conditions specific to a particular body system. Section III focuses on the clinical challenges that face NPs who practice in the acute care setting.

Patient care management is dynamic, and every attempt has been made to ensure that the content presented in this text is up-to-date and is relevant to current practice.

I would like to thank all my authors, colleagues, family, and friends for their endurance during the gestation and actualization of this project.

Barbara A. Todd

Acknowledgments

This book is dedicated to my many patients, family members, and friends, who have been instrumental in my nursing career. I would also like to acknowledge the many nurse and physician colleagues during the years who have shared in my commitment for excellence in patient care.

I would like to acknowledge the many authors who gave their professional expertise and time to participate in this book project. I would also like to thank Linda Scheetz, Sophia Oh Gray, and the Elsevier staff for their expertise and guidance during this project.

BARBARA A. TODD

Contents

I DIAGNOSTIC STUDIES AND CLINICAL IMPLICATIONS

1 Common Laboratory Tests, 3
  Sandra Davis

2 Radiological Diagnostic Studies, 13
  Kathleen Shaughnessy

3 Cardiac Diagnostic Studies, 19
  Mary MacCormack-Suter

4 Pulmonary Diagnostic Studies, 39
  James D. Mendez

II COMMON ISSUES IN ACUTE CARE

5 Endocrine Disorders, 57
  Sandra Davis

6 Pulmonary Disorders, 73
  Anne Marie Kuzma and Karen R. Steinke

7 Cardiac Disorders, 89
  Virginia Buckley-Blaskovich and Carol Twomey

8 Gastrointestinal Disorders, 105
  Kathyrn L. Burg and Karen Campbell Betten

9 Neurological Disorders, 115
  Angela M. Votodian and Jean Dougherty Luciano

10 Renal and Genitourinary Disorders, 125
  Eunice N. Jeon

11   Musculoskeletal and Vascular Disorders, 133
     Annemarie Murphy

12   Hematological and Oncological Disorders, 143
     Colleen M. Harker

13   Health Promotion, 155
     Rosanne Iacono

III   **CHALLENGES IN ACUTE CARE**

14   Nutrition Support, 167
     Phyllis Ann Schiavone-Gatto and Nancy Evans-Stoner

15   Traumatic Injuries, 179
     Corinna P. Sicoutris

16   Sepsis and Septic Shock, 193
     Ruth M. Kleinpell

17   Advanced Cardiac Support Devices, 199
     Mary Lou O'Hara

18   Classifications of Shock, 215
     Ruth M. Kleinpell

19   Sedation Management, 223
     Denise M. Meredith

20   Pain Management, 233
     Catherine Cristofalo

21   Ventilator Management, 247
     Wendy Stevens

22   End-of-Life Issues, 259
     Megan E. Carr

Top Secrets

1. A thorough evaluation of abdominal pain must include an accurate history and physical examination. These assessments are often more diagnostic than radiology and blood laboratory studies.

2. Restrictive lung disease is characterized by a decreased TLC and a proportional reduction in FEV_1 relative to the FVC.

3. Obstructive lung disease is characterized by an FEV_1 that is reduced disproportionately relative to the FVC. The TLC and RV may be increased.

4. Pulmonary infiltrates are nonspecific findings on the chest radiograph and are always abnormal. The clinician should classify an infiltrate in the following ways:
   a. Alveolar or interstitial
   b. Acute or chronic
   c. Focal or diffuse

5. Serum carbon dioxide (CO_2) will be increased with alkalosis and decreased with acidosis.

6. Coexisting infection, inflammation, cancer, or lymphoma may mask iron deficiency anemia.

7. Serum ferritin levels provide a good indication of the available iron stores in the body.

8. Suspect SIADH in patients who have hyponatremia and concentrated urine in the absence of edema, orthostatic hypotension, or signs of dehydration.

9. Common urological conditions such as uncomplicated UTIs, uncomplicated nephrolithiasis, and acute urinary retention can be managed by the primary care providers without a urology consult.

10. When acute renal failure is noted, it is important to diagnose the etiology and to correct the condition before it advances to chronic renal failure and the destruction of functioning nephrons.

11. Infection and bleeding are the most common complications associated with mechanical assist devices.

12. The choice of a ventricular assist device depends on patient history and presentation, patient size, proposed length of support, and the need for either single or biventricular support.

13. C-reactive protein (CRP) levels are elevated in patients with acute coronary syndrome and in patients in whom cardiac plaques are expected to rupture.

14. Cardiac catheterization is the gold standard for the detection of coronary artery disease.

15. Blunt cardiac injury is best assessed by ECG and echocardiography.

16. The Parkland formula is used to calculate a patient's volume needs in patients with major burn injuries.

17. Compartment syndrome is most commonly associated with closed tibia fractures.

18. A midsystolic click is the auscultatory finding associated with mitral valve prolapse.

19. Hypertension control is key in the management of aortic dissections.
20. Ventilator-associated pneumonia is associated with significant morbidity and mortality.
21. Spiral CT scans are increasingly used in the assessment of patients with suspected pulmonary embolus.
22. Poor nutritional status before major surgery is associated with increased postoperative complications.
23. Management of glucose levels can be quite challenging in patients receiving total parenteral nutrition (TPN).
24. Appropriate ordering of diagnostic studies produces the greatest yield.
25. The three most common and serious complications associated with bariatric surgery are (1) anastomotic leak, (2) stricture, and (3) deep vein thrombosis.
26. There is controversy regarding the benefits of off-pump coronary artery bypass compared with the standard procedure for coronary bypass.
27. Hypertension management with beta-blocker therapy is the cornerstone of the medical management of aneurysm treatment.
28. A protocol-driven approach to sedation therapy with a subjective tool to monitor patient response enhances the treatment of agitation in the ICU and may decrease costs, length of stay, and ventilator days because of less oversedation.
29. Hypoxia, hypoglycemia, and hypotension are potentially life-threatening causes of agitation; these conditions necessitate immediate intervention.
30. Anticonvulsants are used to treat neuropathic pain through the inhibition of sodium-gated channels and the potentiation of GABA-ergic receptors.
31. Complex regional pain syndrome (CRPS) is an incapacitating and often misdiagnosed syndrome.
32. Superior vena cava syndrome represents a true emergency in most situations because of the speed at which airway compression can arise and the speed at which failure-like symptoms can arise due to decreased venous return and increased intravenous pressure.
33. The treatment of suspected heparin-induced thrombocytopenia (HIT) is extremely important to decrease the possibility of further thrombosis risk. The most important part of treatment is to stop **all** sources of heparin, including any low-molecular-weight heparins and heparin flushes, which often are forgotten or overlooked when discontinuing medications.
34. As clinicians, we have made a commitment to each of our patients to have two principles as our foremost objectives: (1) beneficence (being of benefit to the patient), and (2) nonmaleficence (doing no harm).
35. The Patient Self-Determination Act (commonly referred to as the Right-to-Die Amendment) requires health care facilities to advise newly admitted patients of their right to refuse or accept treatment should they become gravely ill.
36. Common causes of hemorrhagic stroke include hypertension, aneurysms, vascular malformations, and brain tumors.

37. The most common presenting symptom in patients with an intracerebral hemorrhage is headache. It is associated with nausea and vomiting, and patients usually describe this headache as the worst in their life.

38. Although serum uric acid levels are typically elevated in patients with gout, these levels are often improperly used in making a diagnosis of gout.

39. Compartment syndrome is usually associated with the traditional five Ps: pain, paresthesia, pallor, poikilothermia, and pulselessness.

40. Common complications associated with superficial venous thrombosis and DVT include pulmonary embolism, recurrent thrombosis, and venous stasis ulcers.

41. A decreased systemic vascular resistance is a hallmark of sepsis.

42. The therapeutic goal of resuscitation is to maintain adequate organ perfusion—not pressure or total blood flow.

43. To decrease morbidity and mortality during critical illness, recent data advocate regulating hyperglycemia through intensive insulin therapy (maintaining blood glucose levels between 80 and 110 mg/dL).

44. The role of steroid use in the treatment of severe sepsis is controversial.

45. With sepsis, the treatment goals are antibiotic therapy, circulatory support, and supportive therapies with ventilation and oxygenation.

46. The index of rapid and shallow breathing is a good predictive parameter of bedside weaning.

47. PEEP may compromise cardiac indexes.

48. Treatment of respiratory alkalosis in patients with a ventilator can include adjustment of tidal volume, adjustment of ventilatory rate and, possibly, sedation.

49. *Healthy People 2010* is a national health initiative with two overarching goals: (1) increasing the quality and quantity of life, and (2) eliminating health disparities.

50. Obesity is epidemic in the United States.

Acute Care
Nurse
Practitioner
SECRETS

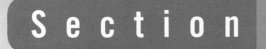

Section I

Diagnostic Studies and Clinical Implications

Chapter 1

Common Laboratory Tests

Sandra Davis

1. **What is the most common electrolyte problem seen in the acute care setting?**

   Hyponatremia is the most common electrolyte problem seen in the hospital. It occurs in 2% of hospitalized patients and is defined as serum sodium (Na^+) level of less than 130 mEq.

   Hyponatremia can be seen in isolation but it is most often seen as a complication of another medical condition. For example, hyponatremia is more common in older patients, who tend to have an increased incidence of comorbid conditions involving cardiac, hepatic, and renal systems.

2. **What is the first step in formulating the differential diagnosis for hyponatremia?**

   The initial approach to seeking the cause of hyponatremia is to calculate serum osmolality. *Osmolality* is defined as the number of solute particles per kilogram of water and is determined primarily by the serum Na^+:

   $$\text{Serum osmolality} = (2 \times Na^+) + \text{Glucose}/18 + \text{BUN}/2.8$$

   where BUN is blood urea nitrogen.

   Under normal conditions, glucose and urea contribute only minimally to serum osmolality.

3. **What are the values for serum osmolality?**
   - Low serum osmolality: less than 280 mOsm/kg
   - Normal serum osmolality: 280 to 295 mOsm/kg
   - High serum osmolality: greater than 295 mOsm/kg

4. **In addition to a thorough history and physical examination, the workup of a patient with hyponatremia should include what three basic laboratory values?**
   - Serum osmolality
   - Urine osmolality
   - Urine sodium

5. What is "pseudohyponatremia"?

Pseudohyponatremia is also called *isotonic hyponatremia*. It may be a laboratory error, in which case it has no clinical relevance. In cases of hyperlipidemia (triglycerides and chylomicrons) and hyperproteinemia, the increased lipids and proteins take up a larger than normal portion of the plasma, resulting in a decreased volume of water and thus a decreased sodium concentration in the total plasma volume. The sodium concentration in the plasma is normal. Plasma osmolality measurement does not include lipids and proteins. Thus the plasma osmolality remains normal. Most U.S. laboratories use ion-specific electrodes to avoid errors in diagnosis.

6. What is the most common cause of hypertonic hyponatremia?

Hypertonic hyperglycemia is most commonly seen with hyperglycemia. Hyperglycemia draws water from the intracellular space to the extracellular space and thus dilutes the sodium. The following corrections for Na^+ can be made:
- When the glucose concentration is between 200 and 400 mg/dL
  - For every 100 mg/dL rise in serum glucose, the Na^+ is expected to fall by 1.6 mEq/L.
- When the glucose concentration is greater than 400 mg/dL
  - For every 100 mg/dL rise in serum glucose, the Na^+ is expected to fall by 4 mEq/dL.

7. What is the most clinically relevant form of hyponatremia?

Hypotonic hypernatremia is defined as serum osmolality less than 280 mOsm/kg and is the most clinically relevant form of hyponatremia. In hypotonic hypernatremia, it is important to determine a patient's volume status as being (1) hypovolemic, (2) euvolemic, or (3) hypervolemic.

8. What laboratory value is most important in cases of hypovolemic hyponatremia?

Urinary sodium measurements are most important in cases of hypovolemic hyponatremia.

9. What are the most common causes of renal sodium losses?

- Diuretics
- Angiotensin-converting enzyme inhibitors
- Nephropathy
- Mineralocorticoid deficiency
- Cerebral sodium wasting syndrome

10. What are the most common causes of extrarenal sodium loss?

- Dehydration
- Diarrhea
- Vomiting

11. **What are the clinical features of syndrome of inappropriate antidiuretic hormone secretion (SIADH)?**
    - Hyponatremia
      - The diagnosis of SIADH is made when the patient is euvolemic because hypovolemia stimulates ADH secretion. In SIADH, the increased release of ADH occurs without osmolality-dependent or volume-dependent physiological stimulation.
    - Decreased serum osmolality: less than 280 mOsm/kg
    - Increased urine osmolality: greater than 150 mOsm/kg

12. **How is the anion gap calculated?**

    The anion gap is the difference between the cations and the anions in the extracellular space.

    Anion gap = (Sodium + Potassium) – (Chloride + Bicarbonate)

    If potassium is used in the equation, then

    Anion gap = 8 to 16 mEq/L

    If potassium is not used in the equation, then

    Anion gap = 8 to 12 mEq/L

    In metabolic acidosis, an anion gap or a nonanion gap may be seen. An anion gap acidosis is usually due to organic acids. Normal anion gap acidosis is usually due to hyperchloremia and is called *hyperchloremic acidosis.*

13. **When treating diabetic ketoacidosis, should the actual or corrected serum sodium level be used to calculate the anion gap?**

    The *actual sodium* and not the corrected sodium level is used to calculate the anion gap in diabetic ketoacidosis. The corrected sodium value would distort the calculation of the anion gap, although the *corrected sodium* value is used to evaluate dehydration. If the corrected sodium concentration is elevated, the patient is markedly dehydrated and needs hypotonic fluids. If the corrected sodium is normal despite a very high serum glucose concentration, then either (1) the patient has maintained an adequate water intake or (2) the onset of hyperglycemia was acute. In this case, the serum sodium concentration will likely return to normal by giving insulin to correct the hyperglycemia.

14. **What is the emergency management of hyperkalemia?**

    Emergent treatments most commonly used to treat hyperkalemia are as follows:
    - Calcium gluconate
    - Insulin + glucose
    - Albuterol
    - Bicarbonate if the pH is normal

    Note that none of these treatments rid the body of potassium (K^+); rather they shift the K^+ from the extracellular space into the intracellular space.

15. How is the fractional excretion of Na$^+$ calculated?

$$\text{FE}_{\text{Na+}}\ (\%) = \frac{\text{Urine sodium} \div \text{Plasma creatinine}}{\text{Urine creatinine} \div \text{Plasma sodium}} \times 100$$

A calculation of less than 1% is consistent with prerenal azotemia.

16. What screening tests should be performed in a patient suspected of having a hypercoagulable state?
- Activated protein C resistance
- Prothrombin G20210A mutation testing
- Antithrombin levels
- Protein C levels
- Protein S levels
- Factor VIII activity levels
- Lupus anticoagulants
- Anticardiolipin antibody testing
- Fasting total plasma homocysteine level
- Factor V Leiden

17. Which blood tests are used not just as indicators of a disease but as true indicators of overall liver function?
- Albumin
- Bilirubin
- Prothrombin time (PT)

18. When alkaline phosphatase (Alk Phos) is elevated, what test discerns whether the elevation is due to an abnormality of bone or of the liver?

The highest concentration of gamma glutamic transpeptidase (GGT) is found in the liver and biliary tracts. Thus:
- Normal GGT with increased Alk Phos = skeletal disease
- Elevated GGT with elevated Alk Phos = hepatobiliary disease

19. How is alkaline phosphatase useful in the clinical setting?
- With biliary obstruction, Alk Phos and conjugated bilirubin are increased.
- With viral hepatitis, Alk Phos is within normal limits or mildly elevated, whereas the aminotransaminases (alanine aminotransferase [ALT] and aspartate aminotransferase [AST]) and conjugated bilirubin are increased.

20. What is the significance of elevated ALT and AST?

ALT and AST are located in the hepatocytes. When the liver is injured, these enzymes leak from the hepatocytes.
- ALT elevation is fairly specific for hepatic damage.
- AST is elevated after cardiac and skeletal muscle injury, as well as after hepatocellular injury.

- If both the ALT and AST are elevated, hepatic problems are likely and the ALT is higher, except in alcoholic hepatitis, in which the AST is higher.
- Order ALT and AST assays to check for medication side effects.

21. What is the formula for the corrected calcium?

One half of the total Ca^+ is bound to albumin, therefore a decrease in serum albumin leads to a decrease in total Ca^+. Serum albumin should always be measured with serum calcium. The formula for the corrected calcium is as follows:

$$4 - \text{Serum albumin (g/dL)} \times 0.8 + \text{Measured calcium (mg/dL)}$$

22. When is it necessary to refer a patient to a hematologist based on the complete blood count (CBC) results?

When approaching the interpretation of CBC results, always assess the three blood cell lines:
- White blood cells (WBCs)
- Red blood cells (RBCs)
- Platelets

If two cell lines are abnormal, it is appropriate to refer the patient to a hematologist.

23. What is the best way to determine a patient's real risk for infection?

Calculate the absolute neutrophil count (ANC) to determine a patient's real risk for infection. If the ANC is less than 1000, the patient is at a high risk for infection. The calculation for the ANC is as follows:

$$\text{ANC} = \text{WBC} \times (\% \text{ Neutrophils} + \% \text{ Bands})$$

24. What is the significance of the reticulocyte count in the evaluation of anemia?

The reticulocyte count is a determination of RBC production by the bone marrow. It reflects the rate of new RBC formation. Normal reticulocyte count is less than 2%. An increased reticulocyte count indicates that the marrow is releasing increased numbers of RBCs into the blood in response to the anemia.

25. What is the most sensitive test to determine iron deficiency anemia?

The serum ferritin level is both sensitive and specific for determining iron deficiency anemia. Ferritin is the major iron storage protein in the body. The concentrations of ferritin present in the serum are directly related to iron storage. Low serum ferritin is considered to be less than 12 mg/L and a ferritin level that is less than 10 mg/100 mL is diagnostic of iron deficiency anemia. When combined with the total iron-binding capacity (TIBC) and the serum iron level, the ferritin level serves as a useful tool in differentiating the various types of anemia. In iron deficiency anemia, the ferritin level is low, the TIBC is high, and the serum iron level is low.

It is important to note that ferritin can act as an acute-phase reactant protein. It may be elevated in conditions that do not reflect iron stores (e.g., acute inflammatory diseases, infections, malignancies). If iron deficiency is present along with any of these diseases, it may not be recognized, because ferritin levels will be erroneously elevated by the concurrent disease.

26. How is human leukocyte antigen (HLA) typing used clinically?

All cells except erythrocytes and thromboblasts have histocompatibility antigens on their surfaces. These antigens determine the immunological identity of human cells. Class I antigens include HLA-A, HLA-B, and HLA-C; class II antigens include HLA-D, HLA-DP, HLA-DQ, and HLA-DR. HLA typing is used in histocompatibility testing for organ and tissue transplantation. These antigens are present in certain diseases so they are used to support the diagnosis of these diseases. HLA typing is also used in paternity testing.

27. At what CD4+ T-lymphocyte count and viral load value should highly active antiretroviral therapy (HAART) be initiated in asymptomatic people with human immunodeficiency virus (HIV)?

The optimum time to begin therapy is not known in asymptomatic patients with disease and CD4+ T-cell counts of greater than 200 cells/mm^3. Although the recommendations regarding the initiation of treatment in this group of patients should be based on CD4+ T-cell counts and viral loads, research supports that the initiation of HAART in asymptomatic people with HIV should emphasize the CD4+ counts more than the viral loads. Guidelines from the Department of Health and Human Services are listed in the following table.

Treatment Recommendations for CD4+ T-Cell Counts and Viral Loads		
CD4+ T-Cell Count (mm^3)	**Plasma HIV RNA**	**Recommendation**
<200	Any value	Treat
>200 and ≤350	Any value	Treat
>350	>55,000	Some recommend initiating treatment (3-year risk of developing AIDS is >30%)
>350	<55,000	Defer and monitor (3-year risk of developing AIDS <15%)

Modified from Panel on Clinical Practices for Treatment of HIV infection convened by the Department of Health and Human Services. *Guidelines for the use of antiretroviral agents in HIV-1-infected adults and adolescents,* October 29, 2004. Available at http://AIDSinfo.nih.gov/publications/pubresult.asp?Finalpubtype=G.

28. **What is the significance of hepatitis A virus (HAV)-Ab/IgM and HAV-Ab/IgG?**

    If HAV IgM is elevated in the absence of HAV IgG, then acute HAV is suspected. If IgG is elevated in the absence of IgM elevation, then a convalescent or chronic stage of HAV is present. HAV-Ab/IgG protects a person from reinfection.

29. **What serological marker is seen after recovery from hepatitis B infection or after hepatitis B vaccination?**

    Hepatitis B surface antibody (HbsAB) is seen after recovery or vaccination. Hepatitis B surface antigen (HBsAG) is seen with acute hepatitis B infection when a person is highly infective.

30. **What is the significance of a normal ALT in chronic hepatitis C virus (HCV)?**

    HCV patients may have fluctuating ALT levels, and 30% of HCV patients with persistently normal ALT levels have histological evidence of liver disease. A normal ALT reading should not preclude liver biopsy examination or therapy.

31. **What is the positive predictive value of prostate-specific antigen (PSA) testing?**

    The positive predictive value of PSA levels that are greater than 4 ng/mL is 20% to 30%. The number rises to 50% when the PSA level is greater than 10 ng/mL. Note, however, that 20% to 30% of men with prostate cancer have PSA levels that are in the normal range.

32. **After treatment of prostate cancer, how often should PSA levels be obtained?**

    After treatment of prostate cancer, PSA levels should be obtained every 6 months for 5 years and then annually. Any detectable PSA is of significance in men who have undergone radical prostatectomy.

33. **What is the significance of cancer antigen (CA) 27.29?**

    CA 27.29 is present on the surface of normal epithelial cells. It is highly associated with breast cancer, although it may also be elevated in colon, gastric, hepatic, lung, pancreatic, ovarian, and prostate cancers. Furthermore, it may be found in benign conditions such as disorders of the breasts, liver, and kidneys, and in patients with ovarian cysts. When levels of CA 27.29 are higher than 100 units/mL, benign disease is unlikely.

34. **What is the major use of carcinoembryonic antigen (CEA)?**

    The major role of CEA is in following up patients for relapse after treatment of colorectal cancer. Measuring CEA is not useful in screening for colorectal cancer.

35. What measurement correlates closely with the diagnosis of thyroid disease?

Calculation of the FT_4I (free T_4 index) is useful in diagnosing hyperthyroidism and hypothyroidism in patients who have abnormal thyroxine-binding globulin (TBG) levels. High FT_4I calculation is suggestive of hyperthyroidism and low levels of FT_4I suggest hypothyroidism. The calculation is as follows:

$$FT_4I = \frac{T_4 \text{ (total)} \times T_3 \text{ resin uptake}}{100}$$

36. What is the significance of the BUN/creatinine ratio?

- Normal BUN/creatinine ratio is 20:1.
- If the BUN rises out of proportion to the creatinine, dehydration results.
- If both the BUN and creatinine rise, kidney failure results.

37. What is the significance of protein found in urine?

Protein should not be found in the urine. Minimal proteinuria (excretion of less than 0.5 g/day) is associated with exercise and concentrated urine in a healthy person, fever, lower urinary tract infections, polycystic kidneys, and renal tubular dysfunction. Moderate protein levels (0.5 to 3 g/day) may be associated with mild diabetic nephropathy or chronic glomerulonephritis. Marked proteinuria (greater than 3 g/day) is significant for lupus nephritis, acute glomerulonephritis, severe diabetic nephropathy, and amyloid disease.

38. What is the significance of leukocyte esterase and nitrites in urine?

Both leukocyte esterase and nitrates indicate possible urinary tract infection. The detection of leukocyte esterase indicates the presence of WBCs in the urine. The presence of WBCs in the urine indicates a urinary tract infection. Bacteria produce reductase. Reductase reduces nitrates to nitrites. The presence of nitrites indicates a bacterial infection.

 Key Points

- Hyponatremia is the most common electrolyte disturbance in hospitalized patients.
- Prostate-specific antigen (PSA) may be normal even in the setting of prostate cancer.
- The patient with anemia should be evaluated to determine the underlying pathology.
- The presence of nitrites in a urine specimen indicates infection.

Internet Resources

Medline Plus Section on Anemia:
www.nlm.nih.gov/medlineplus/anemia.html

Postgraduate Medicine Online: Abnormal Findings on Liver Function Tests:
www.postgradmed.com/issues/2000/02_00/gopal.htm

American Academy of Family Physicians: Special Considerations in Interpreting Liver Function Tests:
www.aafp.org/afp/990415ap/2223.html

EndocrineWeb.com: Common Tests to Examine Thyroid Gland Function:
www.endocrineweb.com/tests.html

Bibliography

Department of Health and Human Services. (2003). *Guidelines for the use of antiretroviral agents in HIV-1-infected adults and adolescents.* Retrieved on March 11, 2004, from http://AIDSinfo.nih.gov.

Hepatitis Association. Retrieved on March 11, 2004, from http://www.hepcassoc.org/news/article43.html.

McPhee, S.J., Lingappa, V.R., & Ganong, W.F. (2003). *Pathophysiology of disease: An introduction to clinical medicine.* (4th ed.). New York: Lange Medical Books/McGraw-Hill.

Pagana, K.D., & Pagana, T.J. (2002). *Mosby's manual of diagnostic and laboratory tests.* (2nd ed.). St. Louis: Mosby.

Perkins, G.L., et al. (2003). Serum tumor markers. *American Family Physician, 68*(6), 1075-1082.

Sacher, R.A., & McPherson, R.A. (2000). *Widmann's clinical interpretation of laboratory tests.* (11th ed.). Philadelphia: F.A. Davis.

Tierney, L.M., Jr., McPhee, S.J., & Papadakis, M.A. (2001). *Current medical diagnosis and treatment.* (40th ed.). New York: Lange Medical Books/McGraw-Hill.

Chapter 2

Radiological Diagnostic Studies

Kathleen Shaughnessy

1. What is a dual energy x-ray absortiometry (DEXA) scan?

This is a dual-energy absortiometry, which uses low-dose radiographic scanning of the hip or spine to identify mineral loss. The results are compared to the range of measurements occurring in normal young adults. Bone mass correlates with skeletal fragility and abnormally low results alert the patient to higher risk of fracture.

2. What chest radiograph findings may indicate a malignant pulmonary nodule?

A nodule with ill-defined margins, greater than 2 cm in diameter, and located in the upper lobes is suspicious for malignancy.

3. What information does cardiac calcium scoring provide?

This electron beam computed tomography (EBCT) scan provides high-resolution imaging of the heart that is gated to the cardiac cycle. It produces three-dimensional views of the plaque density variations. Coronary artery calcification is an early component of atherosclerotic plaque formation. The amount of calcium in the coronary arteries is quantified into a cardiac plaque score. A score less than 100 indicates low probability of coronary disease, whereas a score of 101 to 400 indicates moderate calcified plaque and increased risk of myocardial infarction.

4. Why is video barium swallow (VBE) used for a patient who was extubated after prolonged intubation?

Prolonged intubation may damage the vocal cords and prevent adequate epiglottic closure during swallow attempts. Fluoroscopy records movement of the ingested barium as it passes from the oropharynx through the esophagus. Inadequate epiglottic closure poses a greater risk of aspiration.

5. Why is a cholescintigraphy (HIDA scan) superior to ultrasound in the detection of cholelithiasis?

The HIDA scan is a nuclear medicine study of the hepatobiliary excretory system. Intravenous (IV) contrast is injected and excreted into the bile duct system. Radiation emitted by the contrast is detected by a gamma camera and projects an image of the duct. The duct can be assessed for patency or obstruction.

6. **What is an intravenous pyelogram (IVP)?**

Intravenous radiopaque contrast is injected into the bloodstream, is filtered by the glomeruli, passes through the renal tubules, and concentrates in the urine. Renal function is determined by the length of time needed for the contrast to appear in and be excreted by the kidney. Sequential radiographs are obtained during a 30-minute period to view passage of the contrast through the kidneys and ureters into the bladder. Anomalies of the kidney, ureter, or bladder are identified by decreased concentration of the contrast medium. If the patient is allergic to contrast, he or she should be premedicated with steroids and antihistamines (e.g., Benadryl).

7. **What is the best test to identify the cause of obstructive jaundice?**

Endoscopic retrograde cholangiopancreatography (ERCP) uses a flexible endoscope passed into the duodenum, followed by contrast instillation into the ampulla of Vater. The contrast material identifies areas of obstruction by outlining the pancreatic, hepatic, and common bile ducts. During the procedure, biopsy may be taken or stents placed in narrowed ducts to facilitate drainage and relieve jaundice.

8. **What noninvasive bedside test is used to identify urinary retention?**

Bladder ultrasound outlines bladder contour and can calculate postvoid residual (PVR). If PVR is less than 150 mL, recatheterization is unnecessary.

9. **What noninvasive test should be ordered to confirm your suspicion of renal artery stenosis (RAS)?**

Magnetic resonance angiography (MRA) is the most accurate technique for imaging blood flow within veins and small arteries. Blockage is identified by lack of color flowing within the vessel.

10. **What is the first test to consider when evaluating a complaint of dyspnea?**

The chest radiograph (CXR) is usually the quick, noninvasive test of choice because of the amount of information that can be gained. The CXR provides two-dimensional visualization of the heart, lungs, mediastinum, ribcage, and clavicles. Air-filled spaces appear black, bones appear near white, and organs and tissues develop as shades of gray. The CXR identifies pleural effusions and infiltrates, nodules, bullae and blebs, pneumothorax, enlarged cardiac silhouette, widened mediastinum, deviated trachea, and flattened diaphragmatic domes.

11. **What test best identifies heart valve abnormalities?**

The transthoracic echocardiogram (TTE) uses high-frequency sound waves that are electronically processed and converted to images. This modality examines the size, shape, position, thickness, and function of all four valves, atria, ventricles, and septum. The degree of valvular stenosis or regurgitation can be calculated. Other studies may include the cardiac catheterization and nuclear stress test.

12. **What advantage does a transesophageal echocardiogram (TEE) offer over conventional TTE?**

The TEE is an invasive test using a transducer attached to a gastroscope that is passed into the esophagus. Images have a better resolution because of higher frequency sound waves and closer proximity of the transducer to the cardiac structures. The TEE provides a better view of the posterior aspect of the heart and the aorta.

13. **Can a patient with a St. Jude mechanical valve undergo magnetic resonance imaging (MRI)?**

Yes, because the valve is composed of a pyrolytic carbon coating that is not metal.

14. **What CXR markings are indicative of emphysema?**

The pathognomonic markings include bullae, blebs, hyperinflation, and flattened diaphragmatic domes.

15. **What degree of carotid stenosis noted on the carotid duplex necessitates surgical consultation?**

Carotid stenosis of 80% to 99% with or without symptoms is considered severe and warrants surgical consultation for possible carotid endarterectomy (CEA).

16. **When should endoscopy be performed in a patient with upper gastrointestinal bleeding?**

Patients with persistent bleeding despite blood and volume resuscitation should undergo endoscopy to locate the source of blood loss. Hemostasis may be achieved by thermal or nonthermal modalities. Thermal methods include use of a heater or gold probe, as well as YAG (yttrium-aluminum-garnet) or argon laser. Nonthermal methods include using alcohol or epinephrine as sclerosing agents.

17. **Why is MRI used in the diagnosis of aortic dissection?**

MRI is able to visualize the entry site of the intimal tear, thus guiding surgical approach.

18. **A diagnosis of pulmonary embolus (PE) is suspected in a patient. What diagnostic study is the gold standard?**

Pulmonary angiography is the gold standard test that it provides radiographic visualization of the pulmonary vasculature after injection of iodine contrast. An outline of the vessel wall with area of abrupt cessation provides evidence of PE. Spiral computed tomography (CT) and serum tests of D-dimer are being used more frequently to evaluate for possible PE.

19. **If pulmonary angiography is the gold standard for a diagnosis of PE, why is a ventilation/perfusion (V̇/Q̇) scan often ordered first?**

Cost considerations and availability of an experienced angiographer may prohibit the pulmonary angiogram. A V̇/Q̇ scan requires inhalation and intravenous administration of a radioactive substance to identify areas of diminished perfusion. This test can be performed quickly, thus ensuring prompt initiation of therapy. A normal V̇/Q̇ ratio is 0.8:1.

Key Points

- The chest radiograph may provide many useful diagnostic clues to underlying disease.
- The HIDA scan is a good test to evaluate gallbladder function.
- Upper gastrointestinal blood loss is best evaluated by endoscopy.

Internet Resources

Chest Radiograph Thoracic Imaging:
www.chestx-ray.com

TelMedPak (Radiology Tutorials):
www.telmedpak.com/tutorials.asp?x=Radiology

American College of Radiology:
www.acr.org

Bibliography

Braunwald, E., Fauci, A.S., & Kasper, D.L. (Eds.). (2001). *Harrison's principles of internal medicine* (15th ed.). New York: McGraw-Hill.

Fishbach, F. (2002). *A manual of laboratory diagnostic tests.* Philadelphia: J.B. Lippincott.

Perrier, A., et al. (2004). Diagnosing pulmonary embolism in outpatients with clinical assessment, D-dimer measurement, venous ultrasound, and helical computed tomography: A multicenter management study. *American Journal of Medicine, 116*(5):291-299.

Schoepf, U.J., & Costello, P. (2004). CT angiography for diagnosis of pulmonary embolism: State of the art. *Radiology, 230*(2), 329-337.

Tierney, L.M., McPhee, S.T., & Papadakis, M.A. (Eds.). (2002). *Current medical diagnosis and treatment.* Norwalk, CT: Appleton & Lange.

Wu, A.S., et al. (2004). CT pulmonary angiography: Quantification of pulmonary embolus as a predictor of patient outcome—Initial experience. *Radiology, 230*(3):831-835.

Chapter 3

Cardiac Diagnostic Studies

Mary MacCormack-Suter

1. **What information can be obtained during the history and physical examination that identifies patients at risk for cardiovascular disease?**

   Despite technological advances, the history and physical examination remain the cornerstone of the assessment of the patient with known or suspected cardiovascular disease. The history and physical yield an accurate diagnosis of cardiovascular disease in many if not most cases.

   A detailed and thoughtful history and a thorough physical examination provide the critical information necessary for selecting the most appropriate cardiac tests. A detailed medical history including the past medical history, family history, social history, risk factor assessment, nutritional history, and review of systems should be obtained to identify possible cardiovascular disease and diagnostic risk stratification.

2. **What are the risk factors for coronary artery disease (CAD)?**
   - Cigarette smoking: any cigarette smoking in the past
   - Hypertension: greater than 140/90 mm Hg or medication with antihypertensives
   - Low high-density lipoprotein (HDL) cholesterol: HDL cholesterol less than 40 mg/dL
   - Family history of premature coronary heart disease (CHD)
   - Clinical CHD or sudden death documented in first degree male relative before 55 years of age or in first degree female relative before 65 years of age
   - Metabolic syndrome
   - Polycystic ovarian syndrome (PCOS)

3. **What are the characteristics of angina pectoris?**

   TYPICAL
   - Described as substernal "discomfort" or "pain"
   - Characterized by a burning, heavy, or squeezing feeling
   - Precipitated by exertion or emotion
   - Promptly relieved by rest or nitroglycerin

ATYPICAL
- Located in the left chest, abdomen, back, or arm in the absence of mid-chest pain
- Jaw or neck pain
- Described as "sharp" or "fleeting" discomfort
- Unrelated to exercise
- Not relieved by rest or nitroglycerin
- Relieved by antacids
- Characterized by palpitations without chest pain

4. **Describe the New York Heart Association Functional Classification System.**

   Class I—Patients with cardiac disease but without resulting limitations of physical activity.

   Class II—Patients with cardiac disease resulting in slight limitation of physical activity. They are comfortable at rest. Ordinary physical activity results in fatigue, palpitation, dyspnea, or anginal pain with a slight limitation of ordinary activity.

   Class III—Patients with cardiac disease resulting in marked limitation of physical activity. They are comfortable at rest. Less than ordinary physical activity causes fatigue, palpitation, dyspnea, or anginal pain. There is a marked limitation of ordinary physical activity.

   Class IV—Patients with cardiac disease resulting in inability to carry on any physical activity without discomfort. Symptoms of cardiac insufficiency or of the anginal syndrome may be present even at rest. If any physical activity is undertaken, discomfort is increased.

5. **What baseline laboratory tests should be obtained in a patient with known or suspected CAD?**

   Tests that should be obtained at the time of initial and ongoing evaluation for *underlying risk factors* include electrolytes, complete blood count, thyroid function tests, measurement of serum lipids, and urinalysis. Also, measurement of C-reactive protein (CRP), an inflammatory marker, is recommended, because it is elevated in patients with acute coronary syndrome and in patients whose cardiac plaques are expected to rupture.

   This serum chemistry panel can assess the fasting blood glucose, potassium, urea nitrogen, and creatinine. The complete blood count and thyroid function tests should be measured if clinically appropriate, because anemia and hyperthyroidism can exacerbate myocardial ischemia. Urinalysis, BUN, and creatinine help determine the extent of hypertensive target-organ damage; fasting blood glucose and serum lipid levels identify other cardiovascular risk factors; and electrolyte levels provide baseline values for following the biochemical effects of therapy.

6. **What are lipids and lipoproteins?**

   Cholesterol is a fatlike substance (lipid) that is present in cell membranes and is a precursor of bile acids and steroid hormones. Cholesterol travels in the blood in distinct particles containing both lipid and proteins (lipoproteins). Three major classes of lipoproteins are found in the serum of a fasting individual: low density lipoprotein (LDL), HDL, and very low-density lipoprotein (VLDL).

LDL is the major atherogenic lipoprotein and has long been identified as the primary target of cholesterol-lowering therapy. This focus on LDL has been strongly validated by recent clinical trials, which show the efficacy of LDL-lowering therapy for reducing risk for CHD.

HDL cholesterol normally makes up 20% to 30% of the total serum cholesterol. Some evidence indicates that HDL protects against the development of atherosclerosis.

VLDLs are triglyceride-rich lipoproteins, but they contain 10% to 15% of the total serum cholesterol. VLDLs are produced by the liver and are precursors of LDL; like LDL, some forms of VLDL, particularly VLDL remnants, appear to promote atherosclerosis.

Chylomicrons are a fourth class of lipoproteins that are also triglyceride rich; they are formed in the intestine from dietary fat and appear in the blood after a fat-containing meal. Partially degraded chylomicrons, called *chylomicron remnants*, are thought to have atherogenic potential.

7. **What is the relationship between elevated LDL and the development of coronary artery disease?**

Elevated LDL cholesterol plays a role in the development of the mature coronary plaque, which is the substrate for the unstable plaque. Recent evidence also indicates that elevated LDL cholesterol contributes to plaque instability. However, LDL cholesterol lowering stabilizes plaques and reduces the likelihood of acute coronary syndromes.

The relation of elevated LDL cholesterol to the development of CHD must be viewed as a staged process that begins early in life. Research supports that lowering LDL earlier in life slows the development of atherosclerotic plaque, the foundation of the unstable plaque.

The first step in the development of atherogenesis is known as the *fatty streak*, which consists largely of cholesterol-filled macrophages primarily derived from LDL cholesterol.

The second step is formation of fibrous plaques when a layer of scar tissue overlies a lipid-rich core. Other risk factors contribute to plaque growth at this phase.

The third stage is represented by the development of unstable plaques that are susceptible to rupture and formation of luminal thrombosis. Plaque rupture is responsible for most acute coronary syndromes.

8. **Who should undergo serum cholesterol and lipoprotein assays?**

   A fasting lipoprotein profile including major blood lipid fractions should be obtained at least once every 5 years in adults 20 years of age and older. More frequent measurements are required for persons with multiple risk factors.

9. **What other lipoprotein may contribute to the development of CAD?**
   - VLDL
   - HDL
   - Triglycerides

10. **Describe other blood tests that can be used to assess cardiovascular risk.**

    Elevations of serum CRP and homocysteine are positively correlated with risk for CHD. The mechanism of the link between CHD is not well understood.

    C-REACTIVE PROTEIN
    CRP is a marker for inflammation. Traditionally it has been used to assess inflammation in response to infection. However, there is a suggestion that a highly sensitive CRP is useful in predicting vascular disease.

    The best treatment for a high CRP level has not yet been defined, although statin drugs, niacin, weight loss, and exercise all appear to improve CRP levels.

    HOMOCYSTEINE
    Homocysteine is an amino acid that is normally found in small amounts in the blood. Higher levels are associated with increased risk of heart attack and other vascular diseases. Homocysteine levels may be high due to a deficiency of folic acid or vitamin B_{12} caused by heredity, aging, renal disease, or certain medications. Men tend to have higher levels. If homocysteine level is elevated, then vitamin B_{12} level should be determined; if vitamin B_{12} level is normal, then ensure adequate folate intake rather than modifying the LDL cholesterol goal.

11. **What is B-type natriuretic peptide (BNP)?**

    BNP is a hormone whose release signals heart failure. The heart ventricles release the hormone when pressure rises, signaling a failing heart.

    The BNP test received approval by the Food and Drug Administration (FDA) in 2000; it is currently the only blood test approved by the FDA as an aid in diagnosing heart failure.

12. **What is the role of diagnostic tests in cardiovascular disease?**

    Diagnostic tests can establish or confirm the presence and degree of blockages in the coronary arteries, damage to the heart muscle, enlargement of the heart chambers, congenital heart defects, abnormalities of the heart valves, and electrical disturbances that interfere with the rhythm of the heartbeat.

13. **What is the electrocardiogram (ECG)?**

The ECG is one of the simplest and most routine tests performed. It is often the first test used to follow up the medical history and physical examination. The electrical activity of the heart is monitored through a series of electrical leads placed on each limb and across the chest. These leads act as sensors for the electrical pathway in the heart muscle. The results are printed out on a strip of paper in the form of continuous wavy lines, which represent outputs from combinations of 12 leads.

The ECG provides an initial evaluation of patient with suspected heart disease, detects the presence of old or current heart attack, detects and defines disturbances in heart rhythm, and detects hypertrophy.

14. **What is the electrical conduction of the heart?**

Normally, the heartbeat originates from a specialized group of cells in the right atrium. These cells are technically called the *sinoatrial node*, known as the heart's natural "pacemaker." The electrical signal, which makes the heart muscle contract and pump blood, travels from the pacemaker through the left and right atria to the atrioventricular (AV) node. The AV node then directs the signal through fibers in the ventricles.

15. **What does the PQRST complex represent?**

Each wave on the printout of the ECG is broken into segments designated by the letters P, Q, R, S, and T. Each segment represents a different stage of the contraction and relaxation of the heart muscle, corresponding to the emptying and filling of blood in the atria and ventricles.

The beginning of the heartbeat, when the right atrium contracts and is de-polarized, is designated by the P wave. The QRS segments of the wave represent the contraction of the ventricles. The T wave represents the repolarization of the electrical current and the end of one heartbeat, also known as the *relaxation phase* of the heart cycle.

T wave abnormalities may be associated with K^+ levels. Increased or tented T waves may be associated with hyperkalemia. Flattened T waves or the presence of U waves may indicate the digoxin toxicity more commonly seen in hypokalemia. Tombstone T waves indicate fresh cell death and K^+ being freed in the bloodstream from acutely damaged cardiac cells or new myocardial infarct.

The flattening or depression of the normal configuration of the ST segment is an indicator of permanent or temporary damage to the heart muscle caused by lack of flow, whereas ST elevation is an indication of ischemia.

16. **What is axis?**

Axis refers to the direction of depolarization as it moves through the heart.

17. **How is axis calculated?**

Using the QRS complex leads I and aVF, the axis can be calculated within one of the four quadrants with one glance:
- Both I and aVF are positive = normal axis
- Both I and aVF are negative = axis in the Northwest Territory
- Lead I is negative and aVF is positive = right axis deviation
- Lead I is positive and aVF is negative
  - Lead II is positive = normal axis
  - Lead II is negative = left axis deviation

18. **What are the causes of a Northwest axis (no man's land)?**

- Emphysema
- Hyperkalemia
- Lead transposition
- Artificial cardiac pacing
- Ventricular tachycardia

19. **What are the causes of right axis deviation?**

- Normal finding in children and tall, thin adults
- Right ventricular hypertrophy
- Chronic lung disease even without pulmonary hypertension
- Anterolateral myocardial infarction
- Left posterior hemiblock
- Pulmonary embolus
- Wolff-Parkinson-White syndrome: left-sided accessory pathway
- Atrial septal defect
- Ventricular septal defect

20. **What are the causes of left axis deviation?**

- Left anterior hemiblock
- Q waves of inferior myocardial infarction
- Artificial cardiac pacing
- Emphysema
- Hyperkalemia
- Wolff-Parkinson-White syndrome: right-sided accessory pathway
- Tricuspid atresia
- Ostium primum atrial septal defect (ASD)
- Injection of contrast into left coronary artery

21. **What does a normal adult 12-lead ECG look like?**

Normal sinus rhythm
- Each P wave followed by a QRS
- P waves normal for the subject
- P wave rate 60 to 100 beats/min with less than 10% variation

- Rate less than 60 = sinus bradycardia
- Rate greater than 100 = sinus tachycardia
- Variation greater than 10% = sinus dysrhythmia

Normal P waves
- Height less than 2.5 mm in lead II
- Width less than 0.11 seconds in lead II
- Abnormal P waves may indicate right atrial hypertrophy, left atrial hypertrophy, atrial premature beat, hyperkalemia

Normal PR interval
- 0.12 to 0.20 second (three to five small squares)
    - For short PR segment, consider Wolff-Parkinson-White syndrome or Lown-Ganong-Levine syndrome (other causes: Duchenne muscular dystrophy, type II glycogen storage disease, hypertropic obstructive cardiomyopathy (HOCM)
    - A long PR interval may indicate first-degree heart block and "trifascicular" block

Normal QRS complex
- Less than 0.12 second duration (three small squares)
    - For abnormally wide QRS, consider right or left bundle branch block, ventricular rhythm, and hyperkalemia, among others
- No pathological Q waves
- No evidence of left or right ventricular hypertrophy

Normal QT interval
- Calculate the corrected QT interval (QTc) by dividing the QT interval by the square root of the preceding R-R interval. Normal = 0.42 second
- Causes of long QT interval
    - Myocardial infarction, myocarditis, diffuse myocardial disease
    - Hypocalcemia, hypothyroidism
    - Subarachnoid hemorrhage, intracerebral hemorrhage
    - Drugs
    - Hereditary

Normal ST segment
- No elevation or depression
    - Causes of elevation include acute myocardial infarction (MI) (e.g., anterior, inferior), left bundle branch block, normal variants, and acute pericarditis.
    - Causes of depression include myocardial ischemia, digoxin effect, ventricular hypertrophy, acute posterior MI, pulmonary embolus, and left bundle branch block.

Normal T wave
- Causes of tall T waves include hyperkalemia, hyperacute MI, and left bundle branch block

- Causes of small, flattened, or inverted T waves are numerous and include ischemia, age, race, hyperventilation, anxiety, drinking iced water, left ventricular hypertrophy (LVH), drugs, pericarditis, PE, intraventricular conduction delay, and electrolyte disturbance.

Normal U wave (See the figure below.)

22. What territories of the heart are identified by the leads?

- Anterior myocardial wall: leads V_1 through V_6
- Lateral myocardium: leads I, aVL, V_3, V_6
- Inferior myocardial wall: leads II, III, and aVF
- Posterior wall: reflected in leads V_1 through V_3
- V_1 to V_2, anteroseptal; V_3 to V_4, true anterior; V_5 to V_6, anterolateral

23. What is a signal-averaged ECG?

Another form of electrocardiographic testing is the signal-averaged electrocardiogram (SAECG), or late potential study. This test picks up small currents that are present in the electrical pathway long after normal muscle activation. This test helps evaluate individuals suspected of having certain types of rhythm abnormalities. These currents, called *late electrical potentials*, are generally located in areas of injury and indicate a propensity for developing heart rhythm disturbances.

Basically, a regular ECG is done, but for a longer period of time. A computer is used to superimpose the resulting signals on top of each other and create an averaged ECG, which is then analyzed to detect late potentials.

24. What is a Holter monitor?

A Holter monitor is an ambulatory electrocardiograph. The patient wears a portable tape recorder connected to electrodes attached to the chest for a period

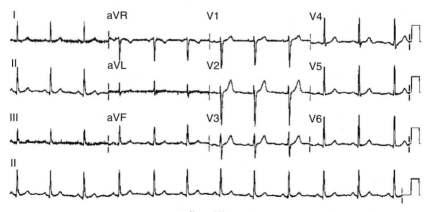

Normal U wave.

of time, usually 24 hours, while going about normal activities of daily life. The recorded data indicate at which point the patient experienced abnormal heart rhythms or the presence ST segment changes. The patient is required to maintain a log of activities during this 24-hour period.

Patients usually push an event marker on the machine when they feel palpitations or chest pain.

25. **When is it most appropriate to refer patients to a clinical cardiac electrophysiologist (EPS) for evaluation and treatment?**

The EPS serves a select group of patients who require treatment for rhythm disturbances. The American College of Cardiology/American Heart Association (ACC/AHA) guidelines are as follows:
- Patients with
  - Sustained ventricular tachycardia (VT), especially when symptoms of hemodynamic compromise and left ventricular dysfunction are associated
  - Dilated nonischemic cardiomyopathy and VT
  - Long QT syndrome who are vulnerable to sudden cardiac death
- Defibrillator patients in order to optimize internal cardiac defibrillator (ICD) settings
- Symptomatic patients with nonsustained ventricular tachycardia and unexplained syncope and with a negative head-up tilt test result

26. **Should a chest radiograph be obtained for every patient being evaluated for cardiac disease?**

Yes. A routine test often used initially after the medical history and physical examination is the chest radiograph (CXR). Anteroposterior (AP) and lateral chest films should be obtained to evaluate heart size, heart shape, chamber analysis, and the nature of the lung fields, especially the vasculature.

The main advantages of the CXR are in separating primary lung disease from heart disease and providing a clear view of anatomical abnormalities.

In general, the CXR is used to define enlargement of the heart or pulmonary vessels; detect the presence of calcium deposits, which may indicate muscle scarring or blockages in the arteries; show any dilation of the aorta; and indicate the presence of fluid in the lungs when heart failure is suspected.

27. **Which vascular studies can indicate CAD?**

Ankle-brachial blood pressure index (ABI) and intimal medial thickness (IMT) studies.

ANKLE-BRACHIAL BLOOD PRESSURE INDEX
The ABI can be considered a diagnostic test to identify persons at high risk for CAD. It is a simple, inexpensive, noninvasive test that confirms the clinical

suspicion of lower extremity peripheral arterial disease (PAD). The ABI is obtained by measuring the systolic blood pressure in brachial, posterior tibial, and dorsalis pedis arteries.

An ABI of less than 0.9 in either leg is diagnostic of PAD, and prospective studies indicate that risk for major coronary events is comparable to that in patients with established CHD. The test is most likely to be positive in persons older than 50 years of age who have other risk factors.

INTIMAL MEDIAL THICKNESS

Carotid sonography measures the IMT of the carotid arteries. The extent of carotid atherosclerosis correlates positively with the severity of coronary atherosclerosis.

Recent studies show that severity of IMT independently correlates with risk for major coronary events.

28. What are the criteria for diagnosing an acute myocardial infarction (AMI)?

The classic World Health Organization (WHO) criteria for the diagnosis of AMI require that at least two of the following three elements be present:
- History of ischemic-type chest discomfort
- Evolutionary changes on serially obtained ECG tracings
- A rise and fall in serum cardiac markers

A new definition of MI has been proposed by a joint committee of the American Heart Association, American College of Cardiology, and the European Society of Cardiology. The diagnosis can be confirmed if there is a typical rise and fall in biochemical markers of myocardial necrosis with at least one of the following:
- Ischemic symptoms
- Changes on the ECG of ischemia (ST elevation or depression)
- Development of pathological Q waves
- Percutaneous coronary intervention

29. Describe the variability of patients with AMI.

There is enormous variability in the pattern of presentation of an MI.

Approximately one third of patients with AMI do not present with classic chest pain. Approximately one half of patients presenting with a history suggestive of MI and who are subsequently diagnosed with an MI have a nondiagnostic ECG.

30. Describe the cardiac markers.

Certain proteins called *serum cardiac markers* are released into the blood in large quantities from necrotic heart muscle after MI. Numerous markers have been identified in the blood. Other serum cardiac markers that are under development include heart fatty acid binding proteins (hFABP), myosin light chains (MLCs), myosin heavy chains (MHCs), and glycogen phosphorylase isoenzyme BB (GPBB).

At present, the standard markers are as follows:
• Creatine kinase (CK)
• Lactate dehydrogenase (LDH)
• Myoglobin
• Cardiac-specific troponins

31. When is an elevated creatine phosphokinase or CK seen?

Creatine phosphokinase is a protein that is released into the circulation from injured myocardial cells. Total CK rises in the blood about 4 to 6 hours after an MI and returns to normal approximately 48 to 72 hours afterward.

Although elevation of the serum CK is a sensitive enzymatic detector of AMI that is routinely available in most hospitals, the total CK level is not routinely used in the United States to identify AMI because it lacks specificity for cardiac muscle. Patients with muscle disease, alcohol intoxication, diabetes mellitus, skeletal muscle trauma, vigorous exercise, convulsions, intramuscular injections, thoracic outlet syndrome, and pulmonary embolism may have elevated CK.

Subcategories of CK are called *isoforms*. Three isoenzymes of CK have been identified as MM, BB, and MB:
1. The BB isoenzyme is found primarily in the brain and kidney.
2. MM is predominately found in skeletal muscle, and a minor quantity is found in cardiac muscle.
3. The MB isoenzymes of CK are predominately found in cardiac muscle, and 1% to 3% is found in skeletal muscle. Minor quantities are found in the small intestine, tongue, diaphragm, uterus, and prostate.

32. Is an elevated CK and CK-MB seen only at the time of an MI?

Elevated levels of CK-MB can reliably identify AMI during the first 6 to 10 hours after the event. However, strenuous exercise, surgery, and other forms of injury to cardiac muscle, such as those resulting from myocarditis, trauma, cardiac catheterization, shock, and cardiac surgery, may also produce elevated serum CK-MB levels.

33. What happens to the lactate dehydrogenase (LDH) level after an MI?

LDH exceeds the normal range by 24 to 48 hours after the onset of AMI, reaches a peak 3 to 6 days after the onset of pain, and returns to normal levels 8 to 14 days after the infarction. LDH comprises five isoenzymes; LDH1 moves most rapidly, and LDH5 is the slowest. Fractionation of the serum LDH into its five isoenzymes increases diagnostic accuracy because the heart contains principally LDH1. However, LDH isoenzyme analysis for the diagnosis of AMI is no longer recommended because it has been superseded by newer, more cardiac-specific late markers.

34. What is myoglobin?

This protein is released into the circulation from injured myocardial cells and can be detected within a few hours after the onset of infarction. Peak levels of serum myoglobin are reached considerably earlier (1 to 4 hours) than peak values of serum CK.

Myoglobin is not cardiac specific and as an isolated level does not reliably identify or exclude AMI at any time interval after symptom onset; it is best used in conjunction with the other common serum markers. However, evidence suggests there is an increased risk of mortality in patients who present less than 6 hours from symptom onset with ST segment elevation and an elevated myoglobin level.

35. What are the cardiac-specific troponins?

Biochemical markers of myocardial injury called *cardiac-specific troponins* (cardiac troponin I [cTnI] and cardiac troponin T [cTnT]) are now being used instead of or along with the standard markers.
- Troponin I is a better cardiac marker than CK-MB for MI because it is equally sensitive yet more specific for myocardial injury.
- Troponin T is a relatively poorer cardiac marker than CK-MB because it is less sensitive and less specific for myocardial injury.
- Both troponin I and troponin T may be used as independent prognosticators of future cardiac events.
- In patients with AMI, cTnT and cTnI first begin to rise by 3 hours from the onset of chest pain. Elevations of cTnI may persist for 7 to 10 days after AMI; elevations of cTnT may persist for up to 10 to 14 days. The prolonged time course of elevation of cTnT and cTnI is advantageous for the late diagnosis of AMI.

36. If a patient has negative cardiac enzymes, does that mean there is no MI?

No. Patients presenting with acute chest pain and a negative baseline serum marker level should have repeat serum marker testing at time intervals from symptom onset. These should be obtained before making an exclusionary diagnosis of non-AMI chest pain.

37. When is echocardiography diagnostic?

Echocardiography is one of the most important noninvasive techniques used in the diagnosis of heart disease. A colorless gel is applied to the patient's chest and a transducer, then a small device that both emits and records sound waves is held against the chest in various locations to produce different views of the heart. Echocardiograms are obtained by reflecting high-frequency sound waves off various structures of the heart, then translating the reflected waves into one- and two-dimensional images.

Echocardiograms are for diagnosing conditions that require knowledge of the anatomy of the heart, such as valve disease, ventricular enlargement, congenital heart abnormalities, and pericardial effusion, and for diagnosing idiopathic hypertrophic subaortic stenosis.

Echocardiography also is the preferred method for identifying intracardiac masses such as tumors and blood clots. It can be used to monitor the effectiveness of treatment for high blood pressure by taking periodic measurements of the size of the left ventricle and the thickness of its wall. Recent studies have shown that left ventricular enlargement diminishes with effective hypertension treatment.

38. What is the advantage of echocardiography with Doppler?

When combined with the Doppler technique, echocardiography can be used to measure blood flow through heart valves and to calculate pressure differences across valves.

Doppler echocardiograms are the best way to determine the degree of narrowing, calcification, or leakage of a valve. The technique also provides measurements of blood flow within the heart's chambers to assess systolic and diastolic function, and blood flow in the major blood vessels and peripheral vessels in the arms and legs.

39. What is a transesophageal echocardiogram (TEE)?

The TEE is a procedure in which the sonar device is attached to a relatively long, narrow tube and inserted into the esophagus allowing visualization of the heart function more closely.

TEE is the only technique that is capable of imaging thrombus in the left atrial appendage with high sensitivity and specificity. It is also used to identify interatrial shunting, aortic atheroma, vegetations on native valves, and thrombus on prosthetic valves.

40. What is nuclear cardiology?

The use of radioactive substances to learn about the function of the heart was first suggested as early as 1927. Nuclear cardiology has emerged into an essentially noninvasive method of evaluating heart disease.

A small amount of a short-lived radioisotope is injected into the bloodstream; then a scintillation camera (also called a gamma camera) is used to detect the radiation emitted by the isotope throughout the circulation. A computer then collects and processes the data, quantifying the information and displaying it as still pictures of the heart.

41. What are the two functions of nuclear cardiology?

The following are the two functions of nuclear cardiology:
1. Assessment of the performance of the heart
2. Assessment of the viability and flow of blood into the heart muscle

42. What is a MUGA scan?

Multigated acquisition scan (MUGA) is a nuclear ventriculogram, which is a type of radionuclide imaging that provides a comprehensive look at cardiac performance including diastolic function, ejection fraction of the right and left ventricles, and localization and degree of myocardial damage.

A MUGA scan is performed by then injecting a radioactive substance, technetium-99, into the patient's bloodstream. The patient is then placed under a gamma camera, which detects the low-level radiation being given off by the technetium-labeled red cells. Because the red blood cells fill the cardiac chambers, the image produced by the gamma camera is essentially an outline of those chambers. It is called "multigated" because a gamma camera takes multiple pictures at very specific times.

A low ejection fraction indicates a weakened ventricle, which may be due to blockages in the arteries that supply the heart muscle, to valve defects, or to a primary problem with the heart muscle itself. A diminished right ventricle may indicate the presence of chronic lung disease, usually acquired pulmonary hypertension.

43. What is a vest scan?

A vest scan is a newer addition in the use of radioisotopes in heart performance studies. This is an ambulatory monitoring system using a miniaturized radio-nuclide detector, worn by the patient and called a *vest*. The test procedure is the same as for the MUGA scan, except the patient wears the equipment for a period of time and is ambulatory.

44. How does one assess the viability and blood flow of the heart?

This is known as perfusion imaging; a radioisotope is injected into the bloodstream and absorbed by the heart muscle as it passes through the heart's chambers.

The basic principle is that healthy heart muscle cells will absorb the isotope almost immediately; it takes longer in patients who are transiently ischemic, and the isotope is not absorbed at all in patients whose hearts have been permanently scarred by a heart attack. Absorption by the lungs of a lot of the isotope is an indication of poor heart function during exercise and is a poor prognostic sign.

In summary, the resulting pictures show a contrast between areas of the heart muscle that are functioning normally and receive an adequate blood supply and those that are damaged and thus do not receive an adequate supply.

45. What is a cardiac SPECT test?

A technique called single-photon emission computed tomography, or SPECT, may be used to obtain three-dimensional thallium images of the heart to:
- Detect individual lesions in the coronary arteries
- Identify the location of damaged and ischemic heart muscle
- Assess the effects of treatment for ischemic heart disease

46. What is positron emission tomography (PET)?

PET is cardiac nuclear imaging three-dimensional positron emission tomography. It measures the metabolic activity of the heart as well as the perfusion of the myocardium. It produces a very accurate definition of areas of the heart muscle that remain viable following MI.

However, because PET is quite expensive and requires highly specialized equipment, it is not used routinely in the diagnosis of heart disease.

47. What is the role of magnetic resonance imaging (MRI) in the treatment of cardiac disease?

A noninvasive procedure that uses powerful magnets and radio waves to construct pictures of the heart in anatomical detail, MRI provides detailed pictures of the heart and blood vessels and can distinguish tissues from moving blood. It is useful in the diagnosis of congenital abnormalities, abnormal growths, and tumors.

As with all MRI, metallic objects can be displaced or disrupted. Therefore any patient with cardiac pacemakers or metallic objects in their bodies should consider other diagnostic modalities.

48. What is cardiac magnetic resonance imaging (CMR)?

CMR is an important evolving technology that can also possibly be used to determine myocardial blood flow, coronary anatomy and flow, and valvular hemodynamics.

49. When should one use computed tomography (CT)?

CT use in heart disease is generally reserved for diagnosing diseases of the aorta.

50. What is electron beam computed tomography (EBCT)?

EBCT is a noninvasive detection of calcium in the walls of the coronary arteries. The total calcium within plaques can be quantified in Hounsfield units for each coronary artery and summed to obtain the total coronary artery calcium score (CACS) for the heart. Amounts of coronary calcium correlate positively with coronary plaque burden. A high coronary calcium score may be indicative for major coronary events.

51. What is an exercise stress test?

The exercise stress test, sometimes referred to as a treadmill test, is essentially an ECG obtained while an individual walks on a treadmill or pedals a stationary bicycle in order to increase the work, or stress, for the heart.

The stress test is used to evaluate complaints of chest pain, establish severity of coronary disease, screen patients at high risk of coronary disease, monitor the effectiveness of anti-anginal drugs, and serve as a screening tool of older adults before they begin strenuous exercise or activity programs. Exercise stress testing has become an important tool for diagnosing "silent" ischemia. Silent ischemia is often detected in unsuspecting individuals when exercise stress testing is performed as part of a routine physical.

Exercise testing can reproduce presenting symptoms. It allows an assessment of the amount of exertion a patient puts forth to produce symptoms, while heart rate and rhythm, blood pressure, and oxygen consumption are monitored.

The goal of the stress test is to reproduce symptoms or the appropriate physical state while periodically increasing the amount of physical exertion. The heart's specific level of function is graded using a scale of metabolic equivalents (METs), which represent the workload on the heart during the exercise test. One MET is the amount of energy expended while standing at rest. The patient's score is determined by the number of METs required to provoke changes.

The rate at which the heart's demand for blood and oxygen exceeds the supply during an exercise test generally reveals the severity of the disease. The ECG component of the stress test allows for the detection of an abnormality even if pain is not provoked. ECG abnormalities are thus a fundamental part of the diagnostic capabilities of the exercise test.

If angina occurs rapidly with little exertion, the blockages are likely to be extensive and the chance of a future heart attack significant. The exercise stress test may reveal the presence of myocardial ischemia, left ventricular dysfunction, or ventricular ectopic activity. It also assesses the cause of angina that is not easily controlled with medication, and it is a way of measuring heart function after balloon angioplasty or coronary artery bypass surgery.

52. What is a stress echocardiogram?

Echocardiography techniques also are applied to exercise testing so that the motion of the walls of the ventricles and other physical characteristics of the heart under stress can be studied.

A stress echocardiogram is done immediately following an exercise stress test. Failure of a part of the heart to contract well often indicates that under conditions of stress, part of the heart does not receive enough blood and is supplied by a narrowed coronary artery.

53. What is a thallium stress test?

The thallium stress test begins in the same way as a regular stress test. When the individual has exercised to peak exertion, a small amount of thallium is administered through the intravenous (IV) line, and then he or she continues to exercise for 1 minute more. After that, exercise is stopped and the patient lies under a scanning camera. By this time, the thallium has traveled throughout the body and is concentrated in the heart, where it is detected by the camera in a series of pictures. This process takes approximately 20 to 45 minutes. The uptake of thallium in the heart may reveal the areas of ischemia.

54. What test should be done if the patient cannot tolerate the exercise stress test?

For patients who are unable to exercise, pharmacological stress testing in conjunction with myocardial perfusion imaging can be undertaken.

IV adenosine (or dipyridamole) produces vasodilation and increases flow to the myocardium perfused by healthy coronaries. This effect steals blood away from stenotic coronaries, creating regional ischemia that can be detected following injection of radionuclides such as thallium-201. This type of nonexercise stress test has proven useful in predicting cardiac ischemic events in patients with chronic stable angina and in those about to undergo noncardiac surgery. Another form of pharmacological stress testing uses the adrenergic-stimulating drug dobutamine to artificially increase heart rate and systolic blood pressure.

55. What is cardiac catheterization?

Cardiac catheterization is the process of inserting a thin, hollow tube into an arterial blood vessel in the leg or the arm. A small incision is made in the leg near the groin, and the catheter is inserted through a sheath into a blood vessel and threaded up the aorta and into and around the heart for assessment of the cardiovascular anatomy and function through the injection of IV contrast.

Catheterization of the coronary arteries, called *coronary arteriography*, is considered the gold standard for selective visualization of the coronary arteries and their major branches. It is the most accurate means to detect the presence and extent of CAD.

At the time of cardiac catheterization, a left ventriculogram can be performed to measure global and regional left ventricular function and assess the presence of mitral regurgitation.

56. What are the common indications for cardiac catheterization?

The following are indications for coronary arteriography:
- Chronic angina with limiting symptoms refractory to medical therapy
- Markedly positive exercise test
- Chronic angina with left ventricular dysfunction (ejection fraction defined as less than 40%)
- Angina soon after MI (spontaneous or induced by exercise test)
- Cardiomyopathy in which coronary disease is suspected cause
- Patients with chest pain who are diagnostic dilemmas

57. What is significant CAD on cardiac catheterization?

At catheterization, coronary narrowing of greater than 70% is considered significant. Natural history studies have shown that the mortality rate of patients with CAD correlates with the number of significantly narrowed vessels, and those with left main disease (defined as a stenosis greater than 50%) have the highest mortality rate. Outcomes are correspondingly worse in patients with decreased left ventricular contractile function.

58. What is a cardiac biopsy?

A cardiac biopsy or myocardial biopsy is a procedure that uses a bioptome to obtain a piece of myocardium for analysis. Myocardial biopsy is performed similarly or as part of cardiac catheterization.

When myocardial biopsy is performed, a catheter is threaded into the heart using a vein or artery fluoroscopy to guide the insertion. A catheter with jaws in its tip, called a bioptome, is then introduced and three to five small pieces of myocardium are removed from the right or left side of the heart.

59. When should a cardiac biopsy be ordered?

This test is performed routinely after heart transplantation to detect potential rejection. It may also be performed when cardiomyopathy, myocarditis, cardiac amyloidosis, or other disorders are suspected.

60. **What are potential findings of cardiac biopsy?**
   - Normal findings with no abnormal tissue
   - Causes of cardiomyopathy
     - Alcoholic cardiomyopathy
     - Hypertrophic cardiomyopathy
     - Idiopathic cardiomyopathy
     - Ischemic cardiomyopathy
     - Peripartum cardiomyopathy
     - Restrictive cardiomyopathy
   - Myocarditis
   - Amyloidosis
     - Transplant rejection

61. **Describe the grading system associated with cardiac biopsy in the heart transplant recipient.**

Standardized Cardiac Biopsy Grading System

Grade	Histopathological Findings
0	No rejection
1 (1A or 1B)	A = Focal (perivascular or interstitial) infiltrate without necrosis B = Diffuse but sparse infiltrate without necrosis
2	One focus only with aggressive infiltration and/or focal myocyte damage
3 (3A or 3B)	A = Multifocal aggressive infiltrates and/or myocyte damage B = Diffuse inflammatory process with necrosis
4	Diffuse aggressive polymorphous ± infiltrate ± edema, ± hemorrhage, ± vasculitis, with necrosis

 Key Points

- C-reactive protein (CRP) is an important inflammatory marker in the treatment of acute coronary syndrome.
- Cardiac diagnostic tests continue to evolve to detect pathological conditions at earlier stages of development.
- Cardiac magnetic resonance imaging (MRI) is useful in the identification of cardiac congenital anomalies and tumors.

Internet Resources

American Heart Association:
www.americanheart.org

American College of Cardiology:
www.acc.org

Cardiosource: A Collaboration of the American College of Cardiology and Elsevier:
www.cardiosource.com

Bibliography

Al-Saudi N., et al. (2003). Comparison of magnetic resonance imaging and contrast echocardiography for semiquantitative myocardial perfusion analysis. *Journal of the American College of Cardiologists, 41*(Suppl. A), 417A. Abstract 1045-1053.

Billingham, M.E., et al. (1990). A working formulation for the standardization of nomenclature in the diagnosis of heart and lung rejection: heart rejection study group. *Journal of Heart Transplantation, 9*(6), 587-593.

Braunwald, et al (2005). *Braunwald's heart disease: A textbook of cardiovascular medicine* (7th ed.). Philadelphia: W.B. Saunders.

Douglas, P.S., & Ginsburg, G.S. (1996). The evaluation of chest pain in women. *The New England Journal of Medicine, 333,* 1311-1315.

Hoff, J.A., et al. (2001). Age and gender distributions of coronary artery calcium detected by electron beam tomography in 35,246 adults. *American Journal of Cardiology, 87,* 1335-1339.

Leong-Poi, H., et al. (2003). Noninvasive assessment of angiogenesis by contrast ultrasound imaging with microbubbles targeted to alpha-V integrins. *Journal of the American College of Cardiologists, 41*(Suppl. A), 430A. Abstract 802-1.

Murabito, J.M. (2003). The ankle-brachial index in the elderly and risk of stroke, coronary disease, and death: The Framingham study. *Archives of Internal Medicine, 163*(16), 1939-1942.

National Cholesterol Education Program. (2001). Executive summary of the third report of the National Cholesterol Education Program (NCEP) Expert Panel on Detection, Evaluation, and Treatment of High Blood Cholesterol in Adults (Adult Treatment Panel III). *Journal of the American Medical Association, 285,* 2486-2497.

Noble, J. (2001). *Textbook of primary care medicine* (3rd ed.). St. Louis: Mosby.

Pearson, T.A., et al. (2003). Markers of inflammation and cardiovascular disease: Application to clinical and public health practice: A statement for healthcare professionals from the Centers for Disease Control and Prevention and the American Heart Association. *Circulation, 107,* 499-511.

Rakel, R.E., & Bope, E.T. (2004). *Conn's current therapy* (55th ed.). Philadelphia: W.B. Saunders.

Regenfus, M., et al. (2003). Assessment of myocardial viability in patients with left ventricular dysfunction using contrast-enhanced magnetic resonance imaging: Comparison to 201-thallium single photon emission computed tomography. *Journal of the American College of Cardiologists, 41*(Suppl. A), 451A. Abstract 1167-1172.

Ridker, P.M., et al. (2003). C-reactive protein, the metabolic syndrome, and risk of incident cardiovascular events. *Circulation, 107*(3), 391-404.

Saeed, M., & Homoud, M. (2001). Cardiac electrophysiology testing—Identifying candidates for therapy. *Journal of Invasive Cardiology, 13*(11), 758-762.

Wayhs, R., Zelinger, A., & Raggi, P. (2002). High coronary artery calcium scores pose an extremely elevated risk for hard events. *Journal of the American College of Cardiology, 39,* 225-230.

Chapter 4

Pulmonary Diagnostic Studies

James D. Mendez

1. **What are the principal uses of pulmonary function studies (PFTs)?**
   - Distinguishing between obstructive and restrictive lung disease
   - Aiding in the determination of prognosis
   - Following the course of a disease over time
   - Evaluating patient response to therapy
   - Assessing disability due to lung disease
   - Predicting perioperative risk in potential surgical candidates

2. **What are the main components of pulmonary function studies, and what do they measure?**

SPIROMETRY

Spirometry measures the volume of air and its flow rate as it is forcibly expelled from the lungs from a point of maximal inhalation. These values are calculated over an entire cycle of expiration and inspiration. The results are useful in differentiating normal lung function from restrictive or obstructive patterns.

LUNG VOLUMES AND CAPACITIES

Lung volumes and capacities measure the volume of air in the lungs at different points in the respiratory cycle. Measurements are made with the patient performing normal, quiet breathing as well as maximal inhalations and exhalations.

DIFFUSING CAPACITY OF CARBON MONOXIDE (D_LCO)

The patient inhales a known amount of carbon monoxide in a fixed time period. The amount of carbon monoxide exhaled is measured. The difference between the amount of carbon monoxide inhaled and the amount exhaled is reported as milliliters per minute of carbon monoxide diffused. A reduced amount indicates impaired gas transfer across the alveolar-capillary membrane.

NOTE: The pulmonary function equipment calculates absolute predicted values for each patient based on age, gender, race, weight, and height. When the patient performs the pulmonary function maneuvers, the absolute obtained result is compared to the absolute predicted result and a percent of predicted value is calculated. Because it is normal and expected that pulmonary function will decline slightly with age, it is preferable to compare the percent of predicted values instead of the absolute values when evaluating the trend of a patient's function.

3. **What values are obtained when spirometry is performed?**
   - FVC: forced vital capacity (liters)
     Volume of air forcibly and completely expired after a maximal inspiration
   - FEV_1: forced expiratory volume in 1 second (liters)
     Volume of air forcibly expired in the first second of the FVC maneuver
   - FEV_1/FVC: the ratio of FEV_1 to FVC expressed as a percentage
   - PEFR: peak expiratory flow rate (liters/second)
     The maximal flow rate of air during the FVC maneuver
   - FEF_{25}, FEF_{50}, FEF_{75}: forced expiratory flow (liters/second)
     The flow rate of air after 25%, 50%, and 75% of the FVC has been exhaled
   - FEF_{25-75}: forced expiratory flow (liters/second)
     The average flow rate of air during the middle half of the FVC maneuver

4. **What values are obtained when lung volumes and capacities are measured?**
   - V_T: tidal volume (liters)
     Amount of air inspired and expired during normal, quiet breathing
   - V_e: minute volume (liters)
     Total volume of air inspired in 1 minute of normal, quiet breathing
     $V_e = V_T \times$ respiratory rate
   - IRV: inspiratory reserve volume (liters)
     Volume of air that can be inspired beyond what is inspired in a normal, quiet inspiration
   - ERV: expiratory reserve volume (liters)
     Volume of air that can be expired beyond what is expired in a normal, quiet expiration
   - VC: vital capacity (liters)
     Maximum volume of air exhaled from a point of maximal inhalation
   - IC: inspiratory capacity (liters)
     Maximum volume of air that can be inspired after a normal exhalation
     $IC = V_T + IRV$
   - FRC: functional residual capacity (liters)
     The volume of air remaining in the lungs after a normal, quiet exhalation
     $FRC = ERV + RV$
   - RV: residual volume (liters)
     Volume of air left in the lungs after a maximal exhalation
   - TLC: total lung capacity (liters)
     Total volume of air in the lung after a maximal inhalation
     $TLC = VC + RV$

5. **What is the difference between an obstructive and a restrictive lung disease and what are some common examples of each?**

   Obstructive lung disease is characterized by reduction in airflow through the airways of the lung. The following are examples:
   - Asthma
   - Chronic bronchitis
   - Emphysema, including alpha$_1$ antitrypsin deficiency
   - Cystic fibrosis
   - Bronchiectasis
   - Mechanical airway obstruction (foreign body, endobronchial tumor, retained secretions)
   - External airway compression (tumor or trauma)

   Restrictive lung disease is characterized by reduction in functional lung volume. Restrictive lung disease may result from pathology intrinsic to the lung itself, from extrinsic factors, or from neuromuscular deficits.
   - Intrinsic
     - Sarcoidosis
     - Tuberculosis
     - Pulmonary fibrosis
     - Pneumonia
     - Pulmonary resection
   - Extrinsic
     - Spinal deformity
     - Pleural effusion
     - Tumor
     - Obesity
     - Pregnancy
     - Ascites
     - Pain
   - Neuromuscular
     - Diaphragmatic paralysis
     - Myasthenia gravis
     - Amyotrophic lateral sclerosis
     - Polio
     - Muscular dystrophy
     - Malnutrition

6. **How are PFTs used to make a diagnosis of obstructive or restrictive lung disease?**
   - Begin with an evaluation of spirometry.
   - Evaluate the percentage of predicted value for FVC and FEV_1.
   - If both are normal, then the patient has normal spirometry.
   - If either the FVC or FEV_1 are abnormal, then the spirometry is abnormal.
   - Next evaluate the FEV_1/FVC ratio.

- In obstructive lung disease, the FEV_1 will be disproportionately reduced relative to the FVC. This produces a reduced FEV_1/FVC ratio, usually to less than 70%.
- In restrictive lung disease, the FVC and FEV_1 are proportionately reduced because of the overall loss of functional lung volume. This produces a relatively normal FEV_1/FVC ratio.
- Evaluate lung volumes if they are available.
- The TLC is generally reduced or normal in restrictive lung disease because of the inherent reduction in functional lung volume. The extent of reduction is determined by the extent of the restrictive pathology.
- The RV and TLC are generally increased or normal in obstructive lung disease because of air trapping. Again, the extent of increase is determined by the extent of the obstructive pathology. Most obstructive lung disease is also characterized by an increased RV/TLC ratio.
- Evaluate the D_LCO if available. D_LCO is decreased in certain obstructive and restrictive diseases that result in disruption of the alveolar-capillary membrane. Significant examples include emphysema, pneumonia, pulmonary emboli, pulmonary fibrosis, and sarcoidosis.

7. How can severity of disease be evaluated and trended with PFTs?

There are currently no nationally established standards for evaluating severity of disease using values obtained during pulmonary function testing; however, the following guidelines are widely used in general practice:
- Normal—greater than 75% to 80% of predicted value
- Mild impairment—greater than 65% but less than 75% to 80% of predicted value
- Moderate impairment—greater than 50% but less than 65% of predicted value
- Severe impairment—less than 50% of predicted value

8. How is reversible airway obstruction measured?

Reversible airway obstruction is measured by performance of spirometry both before and 15 to 30 minutes after administration of inhaled albuterol. Patients may not use short-acting bronchodilators within 4 hours of starting the test. Reversible airway obstruction that is responsive to medication is defined as either of the following:
- An increase in the FVC of 10% or more over baseline after the administration of albuterol
- An increase in the FEV_1 of 200 mL or 12% over baseline after the administration of albuterol

Failure to respond to bronchodilators during the test does not mean that the patient will not derive a benefit from using bronchodilators. If there is a strong clinical suspicion of reversible airways disease, then a trial of bronchodilators or inhaled steroids may be appropriate.

9. What is maximal voluntary ventilation (MVV) and how is it measured?

- The patient is asked to breathe in and out as fully and as rapidly as possible for 12 to 15 seconds.

- The pulmonary function equipment measures the total liters of air moved.
- The result is extrapolated to 1 minute and is reported as liters/minute.
- Decreased values indicate obstructive lung disease or poor respiratory muscle function.
- Poor performance may indicate the potential for pulmonary problems postoperatively.
- The MVV is greatly affected by patient effort. A poor effort will not provide a valid result.

10. **What are the maximum inspiratory pressure (MIP) and maximal expiratory pressure (MEP)?**

    MIP

    MIP assesses inspiratory muscle strength by measuring the greatest negative pressure that the patient can generate against an occluded airway during inspiration. Normal values are generally greater than −60 cm H_2O. Reduced values are seen with impaired diaphragmatic, intercostal, or accessory muscle function.

    MEP

    MEP assesses expiratory muscle strength by measuring the greatest positive pressure that the patient can generate during forced expiration against an occluded airway. Normal values are generally greater than 80 to 100 cm H_2O. Reduced values are seen with impaired abdominal or accessory muscle function or with decreased recoil of the lungs and thoracic cage.

11. **What are the common imaging views for chest radiography?**

    POSTEROANTERIOR (PA) AND LATERAL

    The PA and lateral views are the most commonly ordered views for diagnostic and screening purposes. The x-ray beam is directed from posterior to anterior in the PA view to minimize the shadowing effect of the heart and mediastinum on the lung fields. The lateral view provides visualization of the retrosternal structures that are obscured by bone and vasculature and of the lung bases that are obscured by the liver and diaphragm in the PA view. The lateral view also allows for an assessment of the depth of any abnormality seen on the PA view.

    ANTEROPOSTERIOR (AP)

    The AP view is commonly thought of as a "portable chest radiograph" for patients unable to travel to the radiology department for a PA and lateral film study. The beam is directed from anterior to posterior, so the lung fields are more obscured by the heart and mediastinum.

    OBLIQUE

    In the oblique view, the x-ray beam is directed downward at 45 degrees for the right hemithorax and at 60 degrees for the left hemithorax. This view provides a better view of the superior aspect of the heart and great vessels as well as lung parenchyma overlain by the heart, mediastinum, or bone.

LORDOTIC

With the lordotic view, the x-ray beam is directed upward at 45 degrees to get a better view of the lung apices without obstruction by the clavicles and first rib. The lingula and right middle lobe are also better visualized than in the PA view.

LATERAL DECUBITUS

The lateral decubitus view is generally ordered to better assess free pleural air or fluid that is seen on other views. To visualize the movement of air, the patient is positioned lying down on the contralateral side from the suspected air. To visualize the movement of fluid, the patient is positioned lying down on the same side as the suspected fluid.

12. What is involved in reviewing a PA chest radiograph?

To correctly interpret a chest radiograph, the clinician must be able to distinguish between the different densities that appear on the film. These four distinct densities are (1) air, (2) fat and muscle, (3) bone, and (4) fluid. Air is the least dense and allows the x-ray beams to pass through. Because the air does not absorb the beams, it appears radiolucent, or black, on the film. Absorption of the x-ray beams by other objects causes them to appear opaque on the film on a spectrum from dark gray to light gray to white as the density of the object increases.

A familiarity with chest anatomy is also needed to correctly evaluate a chest radiograph. Each clinician ultimately develops a personalized approach to systematically reviewing a chest film. A typical approach is to evaluate the central structures first, then to evaluate the pleura, the diaphragm, and the periphery of the lungs, then to evaluate the ribs and lung fields in a side-to-side comparison. It is helpful to attempt to visualize a three-dimensional view of the chest in the viewer's mind when viewing the two-dimensional film. (See figure on p. 45.)

Major areas that need to be reviewed include the following:
- *Airways*—Trachea should be midline and branch into the mainstem bronchi and smaller airways.
- *Central structures*
  - *Heart*—The heart should be no more than 50% of the width of the chest. The left ventricle and vessels make up most of the left shadow. The right atrium makes up most of the right shadow. Blood vessels should arborize, or branch out, from the center.
  - *Mediastinum and hila*—The left pulmonary artery is usually above the left mainstem bronchus. The right pulmonary artery is usually below the right mainstem bronchus. If the right pulmonary artery is wider than 12 to 15 mm at its widest point, pulmonary hypertension may be present. There should be no pathological enlargement of lymph nodes.
  - *Aorta*—The aorta projects out behind the mediastinum.

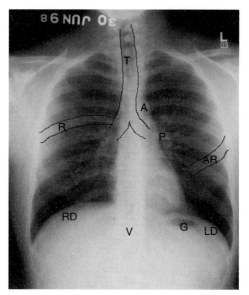

Posteroanterior chest radiograph in a normal, healthy male. *A,* Aortic knob; *AR,* anterior rib; *G,* gastric bubble; *LD,* left hemidiaphragm; *P,* left pulmonary artery; *R,* posterior rib; *RD,* right hemidiaphragm; *T,* trachea; *V,* vertebra.

- *Ribs and vertebrae*—In a normal film, the lung fields should extend over approximately 9 to 10 ribs. If the vertebrae are not distinguishable, then the x-ray beams may have underpenetrated the film.
- *Sternum*—Both the manubrium and the body of the sternum should be distinguishable.
- *Lung fields*—There should be no obvious discrete nodules or infiltrates. It is particularly helpful to compare right lung to left lung to help in recognizing abnormalities.
- *Pleura*—There should be uniform thickness of the pleura around the periphery of the lung. Vascular markings in the lung should extend out to the periphery. If they do not and a thin line with air density on either side of it is appreciable, a pneumothorax may be present.
- *Diaphragm*—The hemidiaphragms should appear rounded. Flattened hemidiaphragms may indicate hyperinflation of the lungs consistent with obstructive lung disease. The right hemidiaphragm is normally slightly higher than the left hemidiaphragm because of the liver below it.
- *Soft tissues*
  - Breast tissue
  - Chest wall
- *Visible abdominal structures*
  - Gastric bubble
  - Liver

13. What are pulmonary infiltrates and how are they classified?

Pulmonary infiltrates are nonspecific findings on chest radiographs. They indicate opacification (increased density) of lung parenchyma. They are always abnormal, but may represent a wide spectrum of disease. They should be characterized as follows:
- Alveolar or interstitial
- Focal or diffuse
- Acute or chronic

14. What is the differential diagnosis for alveolar and interstitial pulmonary infiltrates?

ALVEOLAR INFILTRATES
Fluffy or cloudlike densities that generally conform to anatomical boundaries of the lung reflect the filling of alveoli with blood, pus, or water. Air bronchograms or the silhouette sign may be present.
- Diffuse
  - Heart failure
  - Acute respiratory distress syndrome
  - Pneumonia
  - Alveolar hemorrhage
- Focal
  - Lobar or segmental pneumonia
  - Atelectasis
  - Pulmonary embolus

INTERSTITIAL INFILTRATES
Linear or nodular parenchymal shadows that do not correspond to anatomical structures in the lung represent accumulation of fluid, cells, or collagen within the interstitium of the lung. Interstitial infiltrates are generally diffuse in nature rather than focal.
- Acute
  - Interstitial pneumonia, particularly infection with *Pneumocystis carinii*
  - Interstitial edema
- Chronic
  - Idiopathic pulmonary fibrosis
  - Collagen vascular disease
  - Sarcoidosis
  - Chronic hypersensitivity pneumonitis

15. What are the definitions of common terms seen on the reports of chest radiographs?

Air bronchogram—Normal airways are not seen because they are filled with air and surrounded by air. An air bronchogram can be appreciated when fluid-filled alveoli surround an airway and cause it to become visible on the film. This is commonly associated with an alveolar infiltrate.

Batwing pattern—A perihilar infiltrate in a butterfly or batwing pattern is often suggestive of pulmonary edema of cardiac origin.

Cephalization—Blood vessels are visible in normal lung parenchyma, with those at the bases of the lungs being more prominent than those in the apices because of the effects of gravity. Enlargement of the apical vessels to the diameter of those seen in the bases is often an indication of pulmonary edema.

Honeycombing—Honeycombing is a distinct pattern that is coarse and polygonal in nature. It is representative of end-stage fibrosis of the lung.

Kerley B lines—Thickened parenchymal septa made visible by interstitial edema are known as Kerley B lines. They are seen in significant heart failure.

Pleural effusion—Fluid collected in the pleural space may represent infection, volume overload, malignancy, or trauma.

Pneumothorax—A pneumothorax is defined as air in the pleural space. Lung markings are generally not visible in the periphery of the film where the pneumothorax is present.

Pulmonary nodule—Pulmonary nodules are nonspecific findings on chest radiograph. They are generally well-defined densities that may be rounded or spiculated. They are suggestive of infection, malignancy, or granulomatous disease.

Silhouette sign—A normally visible soft tissue structure is obscured by the presence of fluid-filled alveoli adjacent to the structure. A good example of this is the obliteration of the right heart border by an adjacent right middle lobe pneumonia.

16. When should computed tomography (CT) scanning of the chest be used?

A chest radiograph collapses the three dimensions of the chest into a two-dimensional view. CT scanning attempts to present a three-dimensional view of the chest and aids in defining the location, size, and shape of a particular finding seen on a chest radiograph.

A standard CT scan of the chest obtains serial, cross-sectional images of the thorax. This is done in slices that are 5 to 10 mm thick depending on the protocol of the particular institution. Pulmonary lesions are easily visualized in terms of location, size and density. Significant air trapping can be visualized by also ordering inspiratory and expiratory views.

A high-resolution CT scan of the chest obtains serial, cross-sectional images of the thorax that are only 1 mm thick and performed every 10 mm. This type of scan provides better definition of parenchymal processes, like emphysema or pulmonary fibrosis, than standard CT scanning, but may not capture small nodules that are less than 10 mm in diameter. For this reason, high-resolution images are most often ordered along with standard CT images.

A CT scan of the chest with intravenous (IV) contrast is used to better visualize vascular structures and lymph nodes and to differentiate them from malignancies and other pulmonary nodules. In particular, a spiral (helical) CT scan of the chest with IV contrast is useful in assessing for pulmonary embolic disease.

17. When is magnetic resonance imaging (MRI) of the chest indicated?

There are few instances where MRI of the chest provides more information than a CT scan of the chest. Its utility is limited to precise definition of thoracic vasculature, where required, and in assessing thoracic soft tissue and bony lesions.

Contrast is not usually required for an MRI scan of the chest. This increases the utility of chest MRI in patients who require the definition of a CT scan of the chest with contrast, yet cannot tolerate the contrast dye.

18. What are the indications and uses of lung ventilation and perfusion ($\dot{V}/\dot{Q}$) scanning?

- $\dot{V}/\dot{Q}$ scanning can be used to:
  - Detect pulmonary emboli (PE)
  - Quantify regional lung function
  - Observe the presence of a right-to-left shunt
- During the ventilation portion of the test, the patient inhales xenon gas, which travels to all well-ventilated areas of the lungs. Areas with poor ventilation appear as areas of decreased radioactivity on the ventilation images.
- During the perfusion portion of the test, the patient is injected intravenously with albumin that has been tagged with radioactive technetium. Poorly perfused areas of the lung exhibit decreased radioactivity on the perfusion images.
- Scanning is also performed over the brain in the perfusion portion of the test. If any tracer activity is exhibited in the brain, a right-to-left shunt is likely present.

Pulmonary embolus is suspected when areas of adequate lung ventilation exhibit decreased lung perfusion. The results of the $\dot{V}/\dot{Q}$ scan are usually reported as low, indeterminate, or high probability for PE.

NOTE: A patient may have a low-probability $\dot{V}/\dot{Q}$ scan and still have had a PE. It is important to consider not only the results of the $\dot{V}/\dot{Q}$ scan but also the patient's clinical presentation and lower extremity venous Doppler testing in assessing for the presence of PE. If there is any question regarding the diagnosis, a spiral CT scan of the chest with contrast may be performed. Alternatively, a pulmonary arteriogram is the only way to definitively diagnose a PE.

Many radiologists also report the percentage of ventilation and perfusion to the upper, middle, and lower lung on each side. The total scores from these six lung regions add up to 100%. Although these six scores do not directly mirror the anatomical divisions of the lung, it is useful to evaluate them before any lung resection is done. If the area to be surgically removed accounts for a particular percentage of the total lung function, then an easy estimate of the effect of the resection can be made.

19. What are the indications and limitations for positron emission tomography (PET) scanning?

A PET scan is sometimes useful in determining whether pulmonary nodules are malignant in nature when it is difficult to make this observation by other objective means. A negative PET scan, in context with other radiographic testing and the patient's clinical condition, may prevent resection of some benign nodules.

During the test, the patient is injected with 18-fluorodeoxyglucose (FDG). Tissues with high metabolic rates absorb the FDG in sufficient quantities to show enhancement on the PET images. Highly metabolic tissues include not only malignant lesions but also inflammatory and infectious ones. As such, it can be difficult to say with any certainty that a positive enhancement seen on a PET scan is definitely a malignancy. Conversely, a PET scan that shows no enhancement can contribute evidence, along with other clinical factors, that a malignancy is not present.

PET scanning is used less often to visualize metastasis from a known malignancy and to assess the response from chemotherapy or radiation therapy of a known neoplasm.

20. What are the indications and uses for cardiopulmonary exercise testing (CPX)?

Cardiopulmonary exercise testing is used to evaluate dyspnea that is out of proportion to routine pulmonary function testing. It is used most commonly to distinguish between cardiac, pulmonary and muscular causes of dyspnea, to determine the need for supplemental oxygen with activity, to assess the level of disability, and to evaluate exercise-induced asthma.

The patient performs the test on a stationary bicycle or treadmill using any of a number of standardized protocols that result in a steadily increasing workload. Pulse oximetry and electrocardiograph leads are monitored continuously throughout the test. In addition, the patient must wear a collection system with a tight-fitting mask or mouthpiece and nose clips so that respiratory gases can be measured. Patients should wear comfortable clothes to perform the test and avoid heavy meals within several hours of the test.

Baseline measurements are obtained for 3 minutes. The patient then performs 3 minutes of exercise with no resistance. The workload is then increased until one of the following occurs:
- Maximum predicted workload is attained.
- The patient becomes symptomatic with:
  - Chest pain
  - Severe dyspnea
  - Muscle fatigue
  - Syncope
- The examiner stops the test because one of the following has occurred:
  - Electrocardiogram (ECG) abnormalities
  - Severe hypertension
  - Severe decline in blood pressure over baseline
  - Severe oxygen desaturation
  - Maximum predicted heart rate is attained

21. **What common parameters are measured during CPX testing and how are they interpreted?**

The CPX produces large amounts of data over the course of the test on a continuous basis. The key parameters are summarized as follows:
- Heart rate
- Blood pressure
- Respiratory rate
- Oxygen saturation
- Minute volume
- Tidal volume
- Carbon dioxide production (VCO_2)
- Oxygen consumption (VO_2)

The peak VO_2 is calculated based on the patient's gender, age, and weight. A normal CPX should demonstrate a heart rate less than or equal to the predicted maximum, a normal peak VO_2, and a peak ventilation that is 70% or less than predicted maximum ventilation (ventilatory reserve). If the peak VO_2 is low and the heart rate at the peak of exercise approaches or exceeds the maximum predicted heart rate, there is likely a cardiac limitation to exercise. For a more advanced understanding of CPX, please consult the references at the end of this chapter.

22. **What information is gained from a 6-minute walk test (6MWT) and how is it used?**

The 6MWT is a much simpler test than CPX testing. It is useful to evaluate patients who would have difficulty completing the full CPX. Although it is a crude measure of overall functional status, it is a quick and easy way to serially measure patient ability.

The patient is instructed to comfortably walk as far and as fast as he or she can for 6 minutes on a predefined course on level ground with no obstacles.

Patients may stop and rest at any time during the test. In general, they are not allowed to use an assistive device during the test.

Vital signs are measured before and after the test. Pulse oximetry and ambulatory ECG monitoring are used continuously throughout the test and recorded at 1-minute intervals. Oxygen is used as needed and titrated to maintain saturations greater than 88%. Patient perception of lower extremity fatigue and dyspnea (Borg scale) are measured at the beginning of the test and at 1-minute intervals throughout the test.

The report of the test includes the following parameters:
- Total time walked and total time rested
- Total distance walked
- Average walking speed
- Oxygen saturation nadir
- Maximum oxygen requirement during the test
- Patient's perception of any limiting factors during the test (e.g., dyspnea, leg fatigue)

Normal, healthy individuals are able to walk approximately 2000 feet without stopping during the test. The clinician can readily determine the necessity for supplemental oxygen during exercise. It is common to order a 6MWT before a patient begins a pulmonary rehabilitation program so that ongoing measurements can assess the patient's response to therapy.

23. **What are the recognized parameters for ordering oxygen therapy?**

Current Medicare guidelines indicate that supplemental oxygen is warranted in the following situations:
- If PaO_2 is less than 55 mm Hg or oxygen saturation less than 88% on room air
- If PaO_2 is 56 to 59 mm Hg or oxygen saturation equals 89%, then a secondary diagnosis from the following list is required:
  - Cor pulmonale with documented P pulmonale greater than 3 mm in lead II, III, or A_VF
  - Heart failure
  - Erythrocythemia with hematocrit greater than 55%
  - Pulmonary hypertension

If a patient needs oxygen at rest, then the patient also needs oxygen with sleep and with exercise at appropriately titrated levels. Cardiopulmonary exercise testing or 6-minute walk testing can provide information to adequately prescribe supplemental oxygen.

24. **What are the common causes for abnormalities seen with arterial blood gas measurement?**

- Respiratory acidosis—low pH and high $Paco_2$
  - Hypoventilation
  - Sedation
  - Obstructive lung disease

- Respiratory alkalosis—high pH and low $PaCO_2$
  - Hyperventilation
  - Severe pain
  - Anxiety
  - Aggressive mechanical ventilation
- Metabolic acidosis—low pH and low bicarbonate
  - Diabetic ketoacidosis
  - Renal failure
  - Diarrhea
  - Cardiac arrest
  - Poisoning with methanol, aspirin, ethylene glycol
- Metabolic alkalosis—high pH and high bicarbonate
  - Vomiting
  - Gastric suctioning
  - Diuretic therapy
  - Overdosing with sodium bicarbonate
  - Corticosteroid therapy

25. What are some common abnormal findings on sputum Gram stain examination?

In cases of suspected pulmonary infection, a sputum culture may identify the causative organism. Culture results often take several days to be finalized, although Gram stain results are usually available on the same day that the culture is performed. The clinician may decide to start empirical therapy before the culture results are finalized based on the patient's clinical condition and the results of the Gram stain and other diagnostic testing. It is helpful, then, to have a working knowledge of the types of bacterial organisms that may be seen on a Gram stain. The most common ones are listed.

GRAM-POSITIVE COCCI
- *Staphylococcus* species
- *Streptococcus* species
- *Enterococcus* species

GRAM-POSITIVE BACILLI
- With spores (*Clostridium* species, *Bacillus* species)
- Branching rods (*Actinomyces* species, *Nocardia* species)
- Diphtheroids (*Corynebacterium* species, *Propionibacterium* species)
- Miscellaneous (*Lactobacillus* species, *Listeria* species)

GRAM-NEGATIVE COCCI
- Diplococci (*Moraxella catarrhalis, Neisseria meningitides, Neisseria gonorrhoeae*)
- Coccobacilli (Acinetobacter)

GRAM-NEGATIVE BACILLI
- *Pseudomonas aeruginosa*
- *Haemophilus influenzae*

- *Xanthomonas maltophilia*
- *Escherichia coli*
- *Serratia* species
- *Enterobacter* species
- *Citrobacter* species
- *Klebsiella* species

Key Points

- Pulmonary function testing is a good screening modality for underlying pulmonary disease.
- The PA and lateral chest radiograph is the most commonly ordered chest view for diagnostic purposes.
- Cardiopulmonary testing is useful in differentiating pulmonary from cardiac disorders.

Internet Resources

Virtual Hospital: Interpretation of Pulmonary Function Tests: Spirometry:
www.vh.org/adult/provider/internalmedicine/Spirometry/SpirometryHome.html

EMedicine: Pulmonary Function Testing:
www.emedicine.com/med/topic2972.htm

RadiologyInfo: PET Imaging:
www.radiologyinfo.org/content/petomography.htm

Bibliography

Blumenthal, N.P., Miller, W.T., Jr., & Kotloff, R.M. (1997). Radiographic pulmonary infiltrates. *AACN Clinical Issues, 8*(3), 411-424.

Fishman, A.P., et al. (1997). *Fishman's pulmonary disease and disorders* (3rd ed.). New York: McGraw Hill Professional.

Madama, V.C. (1997). *Pulmonary function testing and cardiopulmonary stress testing.* Clifton Park, NJ: Delmar Learning.

Murray, J.F., Nadel, J.A., & Murray, R. (2000). *Textbook of respiratory medicine* (3rd ed.). Philadelphia: W.B. Saunders.

Ruppel, G.L. (2004). *Manual of pulmonary function testing* (8th ed.). St. Louis: Mosby.

Section II

Common Issues in
Acute Care

Endocrine Disorders

Sandra Davis

1. **What are the major differences that characterize type 1 diabetes mellitus from type 2 diabetes mellitus?**

Major Differences Between Type 1 and Type 2 Diabetes

	Type 1 Diabetes	Type 2 Diabetes
Prevalence	0.2%-0.5% Men = Women	2%-4% Women > Men
Age	<25 years usually at onset	>40 years usually at onset
Genetic disposition	<10% of first-degree relatives affected 50% concordance in identical twins	>20% of first-degree relatives affected 90%-100% concordance in identical twins
HLA (human leukocyte antigen)	HLA-DR3, HLA-DR4, HLA-DQ	None
Autoimmunity	Increased prevalence of *autoantibodies* to pancreatic islet cells and other tissues	None
Body type	Usually lean	Usually obese
Metabolism	Susceptible to ketosis; insulin production absent	Ketosis-resistant Insulin levels may be high, normal, or low
Management	Insulin	Weight loss, oral agents, or insulin

2. **How is diabetes diagnosed?**

The diagnosis of diabetes can be made if any one of the following three abnormalities is present:
- Symptoms of diabetes (polydipsia, polyuria, and weight loss) plus casual plasma glucose concentration ≥200 mg/dL. "Casual glucose concentration" is a glucose level drawn any time of day without regard to time of the last meal.

- Fasting plasma glucose (FPG) ≥126 mg/dL. "Fasting glucose" is drawn after at least 8 hours without caloric intake.
- Two-hour plasma glucose ≥200 mg/dL during an oral glucose tolerance test (OGTT).

Obtaining the same results on a different day or finding another abnormality on a different day, should be done to confirm the diagnosis.

3. **What are the standards for screening asymptomatic patients for diabetes?**

- Screen starting at 45 years of age; repeat at 3-year intervals if results are normal.
- Screen at a younger age or repeat test more frequently if patient has one or more of the following risk factors:
  - Obesity (body mass index [BMI]) ≥27 kg/m^2
  - First-degree relative with diabetes
  - Member of high-risk ethnic populations (African American, Asian, Native American, Hispanic, Pacific Islanders)
  - History of gestational diabetes or delivery of an infant ≥9 lb.
  - Hypertension
  - HDL cholesterol level ≤45 mg/dL, triglyceride level ≥250 mg/dL, or both
  - History of impaired glucose tolerance (IGT) or impaired fasting glucose (IFG)
  - Symptoms of polycystic ovarian syndrome: hirsutism, irregular or absent menses in childbearing years; android appearance and history of infertility

4. **What are the criteria for diagnosing diabetes, impaired fasting glucose, and impaired glucose tolerance ?**

Criteria for Diagnosing Diabetes, Impaired Fasting Glucose (IFG), and Impaired Glucose Tolerance (IGT)

Test	Normal	IFG	IGT	Diabetes
			Results	
Fasting glucose	<100 mg/dL	110-125 mg/dL		≥126 mg/dL
Glucose tolerance (2 hr after a 75-g glucose load)	<140 mg/dL		140-199 mg/dL	≥200 mg/dL
Random glucose				≥200 mg/dL with symptoms

5. What are the important treatment thresholds for treating type 2 diabetes mellitus?

Important Treatment Thresholds for Treating Type 2 Diabetes

Index (for glucose measurement)	Ideal (mg/dL)	Goal (mg/dL)	Unacceptable (mg/dL)
Fasting/preprandial	<100	<120	<80 or >140
Postprandial	<140	<180	>200
Bedtime	<140	100-140	<100 or >160
Hemoglobin A1c	<6%	<7%	>8%

6. What clinical manifestations elicited during a patient interview may alert a provider to a possible diagnosis of diabetes?
   - Fatigue
   - Polyuria
   - Polydipsia
   - Polyphagia
   - Weight loss
   - Abnormal wound healing
   - Blurred vision
   - Increased occurrence of infections
   - Frequent vaginal yeast infection
   - Frequent tinea infection in men

7. What physical examination parameters must be obtained when working up a patient for suspected diabetes?
   - Measurement of height and weight
   - Measuring waist circumference for central obesity (prediabetic metabolic syndrome)
   - Vital signs including orthostatic blood pressure measurement
   - Skin examination (back of neck, groin, and areas of skin folds for acanthosis nigricans)
   - Feet examination
   - Ophthalmoscopic examination
   - Mouth and dental examination
   - Thyroid palpation
   - Complete cardiac examination
   - Pulse palpation
   - Abdominal examination: Check for liver enlargement
   - Complete neurological examination

8. **What laboratory tests should be ordered to establish the diagnosis of diabetes, determine the current level of control, identify the patient's general medical condition, and establish associated risk factors?**
   - Fasting or random glucose
   - Glycosylated hemoglobin
   - Fasting lipid profile
   - Serum electrolytes
   - Serum creatinine
   - Urinalysis (checking for microalbuminuria)
   - Thyroid stimulating hormone
   - Creatinine clearance
   - Electrocardiography, stress test, or both
   - C-reactive protein (CRP)

9. **What is the significance of the HbA1c value and what conditions interfere with accuracy of the HbA1c level?**

   Glycosylated hemoglobin, formally known as HbA1 or HbA1c (shortened to A1c), reflects mean glucose levels for the preceding 2 to 3 months. Measurements are usually obtained every 3 to 4 months for therapy adjustment. Values greater than 8% require changes in therapy. Falsely elevated levels may occur in the presence of uremia, alcoholism, and aspirin use.

   The American Diabetes Association guidelines recommend A1c level of 7% as the primary therapeutic goal for the patient with type 2 diabetes. The American College of Endocrinology recommends a goal of A1c ≤6.5%.

10. **What are the major classes of oral pharmacological treatments for type 2 diabetes?**

    I. INSULIN SECRETOGOGUES
    Insulin secretogogues stimulate the secretion of insulin by the pancreas.
    Sulfonylureas
    - First-generation sulfonylureas (rarely used)
      - Tolbutamide (Orinase)
      - Tolazamide (Tolinase)
      - Chlorpropamide (Diabinese)
    - Second-generation sulfonylureas
      - Glyburide (DiaBeta, Micronase)
      - Micronized glyburide (Glynase)
      - Glipizide (Glucotrol, Glucotrol XL)
      - Glimepiride (Amaryl)

    Meglitinides
    Meglitinides have distinct binding sites that are different from sulfonylurea binding sites. Meglitinides lower both fasting and postprandial glucose, but with the greater effect postprandially. Meglitinides are taken with each meal. They

may be used with caution in patients with liver or renal disease. They are useful in lean patients with postprandial blood glucose elevations.
- Repaglinide (Prandin)
- Nateglinide (Starlix)

II. INSULIN SENSITIZERS
Biguanides
Biguanides decrease hepatic glucose production by improving insulin action at the liver and enhancing muscle glucose uptake and use. Biguanides are often used as first-line therapy for obese patients who do not have renal involvement.
- Metformin HCl (Glucophage, Glucophage XR)

Thiazolidinediones
Thiazolidinediones are useful as first-line therapy for obese patients for whom metformin is contraindicated because of renal impairment.
- Pioglitazone HCl (Actos)
- Rosiglitazone maleate (Avandia)

III. ALPHA-GLUCOSIDASE INHIBITORS
Alpha-glucosidase inhibitors delay absorption of glucose from the gastrointestinal tract, which reduces postprandial blood glucose.
- Acarbose (Precose)
- Miglitol (Glyset)
- Fixed combinations
  - Combination of glyburide plus metformin: Glucovance
  - Combination of rosiglitazone plus metformin: Avandamet
  - Combination of glipizide plus metformin: Metaglip

11. **What are the precautions and adverse effects of the different medications used to treat type 2 diabetes mellitus?**

Precautions/Adverse Effects of Different Medications Used to Treat Type 2 Diabetes Mellitus

Medication	Precaution	Adverse Effects	Benefits
Insulin secretogogues	Risk of hypoglycemia Hypersensitivity to drug Alcohol ingestion Renal disease Hepatic disease Sulfa allergy Diabetic ketoacidosis Contraindicated in pregnant women	Gastrointestinal (GI) symptoms Allergic reactions Hematologic problems Weight gain Hyponatremia	

Continued

Precautions/Adverse Effects of Different Medications Used to Treat Type 2 Diabetes Mellitus—cont'd

Medication	Precaution	Adverse Effects	Benefits
Meglitinides	Hepatic disease Renal disease	Hypoglycemia GI symptoms	Less preprandial hypoglycemia
Insulin sensitizers	Renal impairment Hepatic disease Alcohol use Heart failure	GI symptoms Lactic acidosis Weight gain Fluid retention	Decreases triglycerides, low-density lipoproteins, and total cholesterol Increases high-density lipoproteins
Alpha-glucosidase inhibitors	Inflammatory bowel disease Intestinal obstruction Chronic GI disorders	Flatulence Liver abnormalities GI symptoms	

12. **What is the standard of treatment for overall management of the diabetic patient?**
    - Low-density lipoprotein (LDL) cholesterol controlled to less than 100 mg/dL for all individuals with diabetes, regardless of the absence of other cardiovascular risk factors
    - Blood pressure controlled to 130/80 mm Hg using an angiotensin-converting enzyme (ACE) inhibitor as first-line therapy or an angiotensin II receptor blocker (ARB) as the second choice if an ACE inhibitor cannot be tolerated. NOTE: ARBs do not cause cough or angioedema.
    - Aspirin therapy (81 to 325 mg/day) for most diabetic patients unless specific contraindications are present (e.g., bleeding or hypersensitivity)

13. **What complications are associated with diabetes?**
    MACROVASCULAR
    - Coronary artery disease (CAD)
      - Myocardial infarction (MI)
      - Hypertension (HTN)
      - Dyslipidemia
    - Cerebrovascular
      - Stroke, transient ischemic attack
    - Peripheral vascular
      - Foot ulcers
      - Amputation

MICROVASCULAR
- Diabetic retinopathy
  - Venous dilation, exudate, hemorrhage, microaneurysm
- Nephropathy
  - Intercapillary glomerulosclerosis (Kimmelstiel-Wilson disease)
  - Proteinuria: first manifestation may lead to nephrotic syndrome
  - Microalbuminuria: last occurrence of renal failure
  - Hypertension
  - End-stage renal disease
- Neuropathy
  - Peripheral neuropathy: most common syndrome
  - Paresthesias and pain in feet, decreased reflexes, loss of vibratory sense, loss of pain sensation in a stocking-glove distribution, neuropathic foot ulcers, Charcot's joints
  - Autonomic neuropathy: postural hypotension (major manifestation)
  - Sexual impotence, neurogenic bladder and urinary retention, delayed gastric emptying (diabetic gastroparesis), constipation, diarrhea

14. **What are the commonly used insulin regimens?**
- Single dose of intermediate-acting insulin given daily before breakfast
- Split dose of intermediate-acting insulin; two thirds of the daily dose given before breakfast and one third given before dinner
- Long-acting basal insulin with rapid-acting insulin doses at meal times

15. **What is the onset of action, peak effect, and duration of action for the most commonly used insulins?**

Most Commonly Used Insulins

Types	Onset of Action (hr)	Peak Effect (hr)	Duration of Action (hr)
Rapid-Acting Insulin			
Lispro (Humalog)	5-10 min	$1/2$-$1^1/_2$	4
Fast-Acting			
Regular human insulin	$1/2$	$2^1/_2$-5	8
Intermediate-Acting			
NPH human insulin	$1^1/_2$	4-12	24
Lente insulin (beef)	$2^1/_2$	4-12	24
Long-Acting			
Ultralente insulin	4	10-30	36
Lantus	2	No peaks/valleys	24

16. What are the common causes of diabetic ketoacidosis (DKA)?

DKA usually occurs in type 1 diabetes as a result of stress or worsening glycemic control. Causes of stress include infection, injury, alcohol use, emotional discord, or illnesses such as stroke or MI. An electrocardiogram must be obtained in all patients who present with DKA. Worsening glycemic control may be an indication of noncompliance with a prescribed insulin regimen.

17. What arterial blood gas abnormalities are seen in a patient with DKA?

- Anion gap metabolic acidosis (low pH, decreased bicarbonate [HCO_3^-], low P_{CO_2})
- Compensatory respiratory alkalosis

18. What other laboratory abnormalities are found in DKA?

- Hyperglycemia (glucose often >500)
- Elevated ketone levels
- Hyponatremia
  - Pseudohyponatremia as a result of dilution secondary to hyperglycemia
- Hyperkalemia
  - Initially because of intracellular shifts secondary to acidosis; later because of decreasing serum potassium levels as acidosis is corrected
- High serum osmolality

Urinalysis allows rapid diagnosis because of elevated glucose and ketone levels.

19. How is DKA managed?

- Maintain airway.
- Oxygen.
- Fluids (3- to 5-L fluid deficit usually exists)
  - Give 1 L normal saline (NS) (0.9%) infusion per hour for 2 hours, followed by a decreased infusion rate to complete the rehydration process.
  - When serum glucose levels decrease to between 200 and 300 mg/dL, a 5% or 10% solution of glucose is added to the infusion to prevent hypoglycemia.
  - If vascular collapse is evident, insulin should be given intravenously (IV) at an initial dose of 0.1 unit/kg of regular insulin, followed by an infusion of 0.1 units/kg/hr, with frequent monitoring and titration. As the metabolic acidosis and hyperglycemia are corrected, serum K^+ decreases, so add KCl to the infusion when K^+ drops.
  - There is an *inverse correlation* between serum K^+ and pH. Consequently, *bicarbonate* is given with increased serum K^+.
  - Add bicarbonate only if the pH is less than 7.1.
  - Switch from IV to subcutaneous insulin when serum glucose decreases to 200 to 250 mg/dL. Fluids may need to be changed to D5^{1}/$_2$NS or D5^{1}/$_4$NS; monitor K^+ levels during this time to avoid hypokalemia.
  - The best way to monitor a patient with DKA for improvement is to measure serial anion gap rather than urine ketone levels.

20. **Is the mortality rate higher in patients with DKA or hyperosmolar nonketotic syndrome?**

Hyperosmolar nonketotic syndrome is less common than DKA but has a higher mortality rate. It often goes unnoticed, for example in the nursing home patient with type 2 diabetes mellitus or in the patient with undiagnosed diabetes. Hyperglycemia is usually caused by the stress of illness or by increased glucose ingestion. Hyperosmolar nonketotic syndrome is an insidious process that happens over days to weeks and is characterized by profound dehydration. Ketoacidosis does not occur with hyperosmolar nonketotic syndrome, because there is both some endogenous insulin and sodium present to act as a buffer and to help avoid abnormal protein degradation.

21. **What are the clinical manifestations of hyperosmolar nonketotic coma?**
    - Tachycardia
    - Dry mucous membranes
    - Poor skin turgor
    - Cloudy sensorium
    - A continuum progressing from reduced sensorium, to stupor, to coma
    - Seizures

22. **What laboratory findings are associated with hyperosmolar nonketotic coma?**
    - Glucose levels often reaching 1000 mg/dL
    - Elevated serum osmolality
    - Elevated blood urea nitrogen (BUN)-creatinine ratio
    - Mild metabolic acidosis

23. **How is hyperosmolar nonketotic coma managed?**
    - Fluids are the mainstay of treatment. These patients are usually in an 8- to 10-L volume deficit state. Start with normal saline to correct the volume deficit and then switch to one-half ($^1/_2$) normal saline (NS) to treat the hyperosmolality. One-half ($^1/_2$) NS at a rate of 1 L/hr may be needed for several hours.
    - A workup for sepsis is indicated in these patients.

24. **What are the causes of hypoglycemic coma?**

Hypoglycemic coma is usually caused by excess insulin, delayed ingestion of meals, or excess physical activity. Less commonly it is caused by insulinemia caused by an insulinoma. Hypoglycemic coma must be rapidly differentiated from DKA or hyperosmolar nonketotic coma. Fingerstick blood glucose testing is a rapid means of diagnosis. In insulinoma, insulin levels are elevated with hypoglycemia. Computed tomography (CT) scan is effective in determining insulinomas. Patients in hypoglycemic coma are usually sweating. DKA patients and patients with hyperosmolar nonketotic coma are dehydrated and have dry skin.

25. How is hypoglycemic coma managed?

Patients are given 50 mL of 50% glucose IV over 3 to 5 minutes followed by a constant infusion of 5% or 10% glucose at a rate sufficient to maintain serum glucose levels greater than 100 mg/dL.

26. What is the difference between the Somogyi effect and the dawn phenomenon?

Both of these early morning phenomena are hyperglycemic in nature. The Somogyi effect is caused by a rebound hyperglycemia that is secondary to the release of counterregulatory hormones following a hypoglycemic episode. The dawn phenomenon is the result of an increase in early morning glucose secondary to insulin resistance. There is an increased need for insulin in the early morning because of the early morning release of growth hormone, which antagonizes the action of insulin. The treatments for each are exact opposites.

27. What are the treatments for the Somogyi effect and the dawn phenomenon?

Treatments for Somogyi Effect and Dawn Phenomenon	
Disorder	**Treatment**
Somogyi effect	Take NPH or Lente insulin before bed, instead of before dinner. Switch to a longer acting preparation. Measure 3 AM glucose (it will usually be decreased).
Dawn phenomenon	Increase the insulin dosage.

28. What is the insulin resistance syndrome (IRS)?

IRS is also known as *dysmetabolic syndrome* and as *syndrome X*. It has also been associated with polycystic ovarian syndrome.

IRS results from a reduced sensitivity to the effects of insulin on glucose uptake by insulin-sensitive tissues. About 50% of a patient's insulin resistance is due to genetic factors. It is made worse by age, inactivity, and the development of obesity. Other environmental factors that increase insulin resistance are cigarette smoking, infections, and cancers. IRS, also known as the *dysmetabolic syndrome,* is characterized by hypertension, dyslipidemia, glucose intolerance, and visceral obesity. Insulin resistance is an independent risk factor for ischemic heart disease.

29. **What landmark studies demonstrated the importance of intensive diabetes treatment by keeping blood glucose as close to normal as possible to avoid long-term complications?**

The results from the 1993 Diabetes Control and Complications Trial (DCCT) demonstrated that near-normalization of blood glucose levels in individuals with type 1 diabetes significantly delays the onset and slows the progression of complications associated with the disease.

The 1998 United Kingdom Prospective Diabetes Study (UKPDS) demonstrated the benefits of near-normalization of blood glucose in type 2 diabetes intended to decrease associated complications.

30. **What are the causes of Cushing's syndrome?**

The most common cause of Cushing's syndrome is iatrogenic as a result of the administration of large doses of steroids for the treatment of a primary disease. Cushing's syndrome may also be caused by increased levels of pituitary adreno-corticotropic hormone (ACTH), leading to bilateral adrenal hyperplasia, also known as *Cushing's disease.* Adrenal adenoma or carcinoma as well as oat cell carcinoma of the lung may cause Cushing's syndrome. Ectopic ACTH production by tumors may also cause Cushing's syndrome.

31. **What are the clinical manifestations associated with Cushing's disease?**
   - "Cushingoid" appearance (central or truncal obesity) caused by excess cortisol secretion on fat distribution, facial plethora, hirsutism (in women), striae, and menstrual disorders
   - Hypertension caused by vascular effects of cortisol and sodium retention
   - Decreased glucose tolerance, polyuria, and polydipsia caused by increased hepatic gluconeogenesis and decreased peripheral glucose use
   - Muscle wasting and weakness (large abdomen, but disproportionately thin arms and legs) caused by catabolic changes
   - Osteoporosis caused by increased bone catabolism
   - Easy bruising caused by enhanced capillary fragility
   - Depression (psychiatric disturbances)
   - Back pain
   - Acne, oily skin
   - Renal calculi
   - Heart failure
   - Acanthosis nigricans (hyperpigmentation)

32. **What laboratory findings and diagnostic tests are used to establish Cushing's syndrome and Cushing's disease?**
   - 24-hour urinary free cortisol excretion rate
   - ACTH measurement
   - Standard low-dose dexamethasone suppression test

- High-dose dexamethasone suppression test
- CT scan of the adrenals
- CT scan of the head
- Serum thyroid-stimulating hormone (TSH) level to exclude thyroid tumor

33. What are the treatment options for Cushing's syndrome?

- Transsphenoidal surgery and radiation of pituitary tumor
- Surgical resection of adrenal tumor

34. What are the clinical manifestations of an adrenal crisis?

- Fever
- Vomiting
- Abdominal pain
- Altered mental status
- Vascular collapse, if not treated

An addisonian crisis or adrenal crisis is an acute, life-threatening complication of Addison's disease. In an adrenal crisis, the manifestations of adrenal insufficiency are exaggerated.

35. What is Addison's disease?

Addison's disease is severe or total deficiency of the hormones made in the adrenal cortex (cortisol and aldosterone).

36. What is the treatment for an adrenal crisis?

The treatment for adrenal crisis is immediate IV administration of 100 mg of cortisol over 5 to 10 minutes. This should be followed by an additional 300 mg over the next 24 hours. IV saline is also needed. If hypotension and volume depletion persist, mineralocorticoid replacement should be provided.

37. What are the causes of diabetes insipidus (DI)?

- Inadequate arginine vasopressin (antidiuretic hormone [ADH]) results in DI. Etiology is either central or neurogenic. Causes of central DI include head trauma (most commonly seen in intensive care units), brain tumors, neurosurgical procedures, and injury to the hypothalamic-pituitary area. Nephrogenic DI is the result of renal unresponsiveness to ADH.
- Many medications cause DI, such as lithium, demeclocycline, and cisplatin.
- Gestation, pre-eclampsia, or toxemia of pregnancy is also a cause of DI.

38. What are the laboratory findings in DI?

- Low urine osmolality (<300 mOsm/kg)
- Specific gravity less than 1.010

- High or normal serum osmolality (≥280 mOsm/kg)
- In psychogenic polydipsia, serum osmolality is <280 mOsm/kg because of excessive water intake
- Hypernatremia
- Elevated BUN/creatinine

39. What is the hallmark of syndrome of inappropriate antidiuretic hormone secretion (SIADH)?

Hyponatremia is the hallmark of SIADH. SIADH should be expected in patients with hyponatremia and a concentrated urine (osmolality >300 mmol/kg) in the absence of edema, orthostatic hypotension, and features of dehydration.

40. What is the treatment of SIADH?

- Restriction of free water
- Agents to counter the action of ADH: lithium carbonate or demeclocycline

41. Which treatments should be avoided in SIADH?

- Diuretics
- Hypertonic saline solutions

42. What are the potential causes of a thyroid nodule?

A patient who presents with a thyroid nodule may have true adenoma or carcinoma, but he or she may otherwise have cysts, colloid nodules, hemorrhagic necrotic tissue, or areas of chronic thyroiditis. Thyroid nodules are present in 1% of patients in the 20-year-old age-group and in 5% of patients in the 60-year-old age-group. These nodules are found to be cancerous in 5% of the cases.

43. How are thyroid nodules diagnosed?

It is important to make the diagnosis based on (1) the patient's history, which includes a thorough risk assessment for the development of thyroid nodules or cancer, (2) physical examination, and (3) laboratory and diagnostic findings.

44. What diagnostic findings may suggest thyroid malignancy?

- History of radiation treatment to the head or neck in childhood
- Male gender
  - A higher percentage of nodules are malignant in men, but nodules are much more common in women.
- Younger age
  - A higher percentage of nodules are malignant in younger individuals, but nodules are more common in older individuals.

- Progression of disease
  - Malignancy is less likely in the following cases:
    There are multiple nodules or the nodule is less than 1 cm in diameter.
    The nodule disappears after aspiration of cyst fluid.
    The nodule is visible as warm or hot on scintiscan.
    The nodule shrinks with suppressive therapy.
  - Malignancy is more likely in the following cases:
    The nodule is fixed in place and no movement occurs when swallowing on physical examination.
    There is recent or continued growth of a nodule despite treatment with L-thyroxine.
    There is firm consistency of the nodule, irregularity of the nodule, or regional lymph node enlargement.

45. How common is primary hyperparathyroidism?

Primary hyperparathyroidism is common. It is especially common in middle-aged and older women. A single parathyroid adenoma causes 80% to 90% of cases and hyperplasia of all four glands occurs in 10% to 20% of cases. Parathyroid carcinoma is a rare cause. Primary hyperparathyroidism results from the oversecretion of parathyroid hormone, which in turn causes hypercalcemia.

46. What is the most common cause of hypoparathyroidism?

Surgical removal of the parathyroid glands is the most common cause of hypoparathyroidism. Surgical removal may be unavoidable as a result of radical neck dissection for cancer or it may be a rare complication of subtotal thyroidectomy. Idiopathic hypoparathyroidism of autoimmune etiology is less common.

47. What are the various types of thyroiditis?

- Hashimoto's thyroiditis or chronic autoimmune thyroiditis. Antithyroid antibodies are present in most patients.
- Subacute thyroiditis, which is generally considered to be viral. Viruses such as mumps and Coxsackievirus have been suspected.
- Painless thyroiditis, also referred to as *postpartum thyroiditis*. It is a transient, self-limited hyperthyroidism with thyroid gland enlargement and no thyroid pain or tenderness. A low radioactive iodine uptake is the most useful finding for distinguishing painless thyroiditis from Graves' disease.

48. Should a patient with subclinical hypothyroidism be treated with thyroid hormone?

In subclinical hypothyroidism the serum TSH is elevated but the serum free T_4 is normal, not decreased as expected. The decision to treat should be made on an individual basis. Factors that weigh more toward treating are (1) symptoms of hypothyroidism, (2) presence of antithyroid antibodies, and (3) greater degree of TSH elevation.

🔑 Key Points

- Insulin resistance is characterized by central obesity, hyperinsulinemia, hypertriglyceridemia, low LDL cholesterol, hypertension, and glucose intolerance.
- The presence of diabetes mellitus is considered a coronary heart disease (CHD) risk equivalent and patients with diabetes are considered to have CHD even in the absence of symptoms.
- Patients taking metformin should be monitored closely for lactic acidosis.
- Cushing's syndrome is commonly caused by administration of high-dose steroids.

Internet Resources

American Diabetes Association Homepage:
www.diabetes.org

National Institute of Diabetes and Digestive and Kidney Diseases:
www.niddk.nih.gov

Endocrine Disorders and Endocrine Surgery:
www.endocrineweb.com

Bibliography

American Association of Clinical Endocrinologists. (2002). Medical guidelines for the management of diabetes mellitus: The AACE system of intensive diabetes self-management—2002 update. *Endocrine Practice, 18*(Suppl. 1), 41-82.

American College of Endocrinology. (2003). Position statement on the insulin resistance syndrome. *Endocrine Practice, 9*(3), 236-239.

American Diabetes Association. (2002). Position statement: Screening for diabetes. *Diabetes Care, 25*(Suppl.), S21-S24.

Barkley, T., Myers, C. (2001). *Practice guidelines for acute care nurse practitioners.* Philadelphia: W.B. Saunders.

Ford, E.S., Giles, W.H., & Dietz, W.H. (2002). Prevalence of the metabolic syndrome among US adults: Findings from the third National Health and Nutrition Examination Survey. *Journal of the American Medical Association, 287,* 356-359.

Mittman, B. (2002). *Nail the boards.* Valley Stream, NY: Frontrunners Board Review.

Myers, A. (2001). *Medicine* (4th ed.). Philadelphia: Lippincott Williams & Wilkins.

National Cholesterol Education Program. (2001). Executive summary of the Third Report of the National Cholesterol Education Program (NCEP) Expert Panel on Detection, Evaluation, and Treatment of High Blood Cholesterol in Adults (Adult Treatment Panel III). *Journal of the American Medical Association, 285,* 2486-2497.

Nirula, R. (1997). *High-yield internal medicine.* Philadelphia: Lippincott Williams & Wilkins.

Chapter 6

Pulmonary Disorders

Anne Marie Kuzma and Karen R. Steinke

1. What is the major muscle of respiration?

The diaphragm is the major muscle of respiration.

2. What are the accessory muscles of respiration?

- Scalenes
- Sternocleidomastoids

3. What is the most common cause of community-acquired pneumonia?

The most common organism responsible for approximately 50% of acute community-acquired pneumonia is *Streptococcus pneumoniae*. In older adults, community-acquired pneumonia is frequently caused by aerobic gram-negative bacilli as well as by *Staphylococcus aureus*. This may be due to increased colonization of the pharynx by gram-negative rods secondary to a serious underlying disease, prior antibiotic therapy, and a decrease in overall physical activity. During winter, older adults are at risk for influenza pneumonia. The clinical presentation of community-acquired pneumonia varies with the cause and the comorbidities of the person affected.

4. Describe the clinical course associated with pneumonia.

Pneumonia due to pyogenic organisms such as *Streptococcal pneumoniae, Staphylococcus aureus,* or *Haemophilus influenzae* usually present with a fever, productive cough, chest pain, and shortness of breath. The respiratory rate is increased and the patient may need to use accessory muscles. The clinical picture varies depending on the age of the patient, the immune state, and the type of microorganism. The patient with bacterial pneumonia manifests respiratory distress and often needs to be observed in an intensive care unit (ICU). The physical examination of the affected lung shows evidence of consolidation, increased vocal fremitus, and dullness to percussion, crackles, whispered pectoriloquy, and egophony.

5. What is the incidence of pneumonia-associated mortality?

An estimated 50,000 patients die of pneumonia each year. About 5% of all patients with pneumonia die. If bacteremia is also present, the rate increases to 20%.

6. **What are the risk factors associated with mortality in the patient with pneumonia?**

   Older age and underlying medical conditions such as previous splenectomy, cirrhosis, chronic obstructive pulmonary disease (COPD), immunodeficiency syndromes, and malignancies are strongly associated with increased mortality. If leukopenia, jaundice, extrapulmonary complications, and involvement of three or more lobes of the lung are seen on the chest radiograph, the prognosis is poor.

7. **What is the most common type of community-acquired pneumonia?**

   Pneumococcal pneumonia is the most common type of community-acquired pneumonia.

8. **What diagnostic tests are usually ordered in a patient with suspected pneumonia?**
   - Chest radiograph
   - Sputum cultures
   - Blood cultures
   - Complete blood count

9. **What is the frequency of nosocomial pneumonia?**

   Nosocomial pneumonia is the second leading hospital-acquired infection. Pneumonia develops in nearly 1% of patients admitted to the hospital. About one third of these patients die. Pneumonia develops in 60% of ICU patients. The most common microorganisms are gram-negative bacilli and *Staphylococcus aureus*. The microorganism responsible for nosocomial pneumonia infections varies between institutions.

10. **What hospital variables may predispose patients to pneumonia?**
    - Aspiration
    - Mechanical ventilation
    - Feeding tubes
    - Sedation
    - Colonization of the gastrointestinal tract, which may be associated with decreased gastric acidity from the use of histamine blockers

11. **Should empirical antibiotics be used to prevent nosocomial pneumonia?**

    Because of the high mortality rate associated with nosocomial pneumonia and the presence of resistant organisms in most hospitals, the use of broad-spectrum antibiotics is begun as soon as pneumonia is suspected. Once an organism is identified, the antibiotic can be targeted to the pathogen. Patients who have been hospitalized for more than 3 days and are seriously ill are likely to be colonized with resistant gram-negative organisms.

12. **What microorganisms are seen most frequently in patients on mechanical ventilation?**

Pseudomonas and *Enterobacter* species are the organisms seen most frequently in patients on mechanical ventilation.

13. **What clinical signs are associated with atypical pneumonia?**
    - Low-grade fever
    - Nonproductive cough
    - Myalgia

14. **What are the common causes of atypical pneumonia?**
    - *Mycoplasma*
    - Viruses
    - *Chlamydia*

15. **What is a solitary pulmonary nodule (SPN)?**

SPN is a radiographic finding of a small ($\leq$4 cm) round density surrounded by normal lung tissue without intrathoracic adenopathy or associated atelectasis. The nodule may be calcified or noncalcified, and the border may be irregular or sharp.

16. **What are the causes of SPN?**

The most common cause of SPN is granuloma. These may be due to prior lung infections, such as histoplasmosis and tuberculosis. Neoplasms are either bronchogenic or carcinogenic, or they metastasize from extrathoracic malignancies. Bronchogenic carcinoma accounts for approximately one third of all SPNs.

17. **How is an SPN diagnosed?**
    - Physical examination
    - Induced sputum with hypertonic saline
    - Chest computed tomography (CT) scan
    - Biopsy

18. **Define chronic obstructive pulmonary disease (COPD).**

COPD is a disease characterized by airflow limitations. Disease states include emphysema and chronic bronchitis.

19. **What is the incidence of COPD?**

Approximately 14 million people in the United States have COPD; emphysema is the fourth leading cause of death.

20. **What is the correlation between cigarette smoking and COPD?**

   Cigarette smoking is the leading cause of emphysema. Cigarette smoking is thought to induce an imbalance between protease and antiprotease in the lungs. This interaction increases the elastase activity and destruction of the elastic fibers of the alveolar walls. The benefits of smoking cessation are well established. In younger smokers (35 years of age) with mild COPD, the forced expiratory volume in 1 second (FEV_1) returns to normal after the patient stops smoking. In older patients, cessation slows the progress of the disease but does not eliminate the disease.

21. **Describe the physiological effects of COPD.**

   Airflow limitations caused by the airway lumens occluded by excessive and tenacious secretions are common in emphysema. The contraction of airways smooth muscles and bronchial wall edema and inflammation decrease the luminal diameters of the airways. As the parenchyma of the lung is destroyed, the tethering forces exerted on the airway lumens are diminished. Moderate-sized airways become floppy during forced expiration. Pulmonary mechanics, including expiratory flow rates and volumes, are diminished during the prolonged expiration time, which prevents complete emptying of the affected alveoli. Lung volumes are increased, which causes the diaphragm to be flattened. In patients with COPD, the work of breathing is increased due to the increase in airway resistance and the altered respiratory muscle mechanics.

22. **What are the two classifications of patients with COPD?**
   - Pink puffer
   - Blue bloater

23. **Describe the difference between the pink puffer and the blue bloater.**

   This classification of COPD patients is used to define the underlying process. This classification has become less useful because there is a significant amount of overlap and few patients fall exclusively into either subset. A pink puffer is tachypneic with labored respirations and pursed lip breathing. Arterial oxygenation is usually preserved. A blue bloater is a patient who appears chronically cyanotic (arterial hypoxemia), is hypercapnic, has leg swelling, and has right-sided heart failure. Patients tend to be obese and often produce mucus on a regular basis. The blue bloater is associated with chronic bronchitis and pink puffers are associated with emphysema.

24. **What are common physical examination findings in patients with COPD?**
   - Diminished breath sounds
   - Expiratory wheezing
   - Prolonged expiratory phase
   - Increased anteroposterior diameter of the chest wall
   - Limited excursion of the diaphragm
   - Signs of right-sided heart failure, if the patient is hypoxemic

25. **Describe the treatment protocol for a patient admitted with acute exacerbation of COPD.**

Patients admitted with shortness of breath related to emphysema need to be monitored for respiratory failure. Hospitalized patients should be switched from meter-dosed inhalers to nebulizers. Bronchodilator dosage needs to be intensified during exacerbation. Nebulized treatments of albuterol, a short-acting bronchodilator, are increased to 5 to 7.5 mg every 2 to 3 hours. Treatments of ipratropium bromide, an anticholinergic agent that decreases vagal tone, inhibits smooth muscle contraction, and decreases secretions, should be administered every 6 hours. It is important to ensure that all bronchodilators are given as prescribed to prevent excessive hyperinflation.

Theophylline may be used long term or started during an exacerbation. The mechanism in which theophylline works is unknown, but this agent decreases dyspnea and airway obstruction. Optimal bronchodilator effects may occur in the low therapeutic range (5 to 15 mg/dL).

Pulse-dose steroids are started in patients with exacerbation. As the patient's breathlessness improves, the steroid dose can be decreased and tapered, as can the bronchodilators.

Intubation should be avoided if possible. Noninvasive positive-pressure ventilation can be used to decrease breathlessness, improve oxygenation, and lower carbon dioxide. Vapotherm, high-flow humidified oxygen, has been shown to decrease breathlessness during acute exacerbation.

26. **What is the natural progression of COPD?**

The natural progression of emphysema is often correlated to the FEV_1. Median survival is approximately 10 years when FEV_1 is 1.4 L, 4 years when FEV_1 is 1 L, and less than 2 years when FEV_1 is 0.5 L.

27. **What is tuberculosis (TB)?**

TB refers to a disease caused by *Mycobacterium tuberculosis,* a nonmotile bacillus. TB is a major world health problem associated with an estimated 8 million new cases and approximately 3 million deaths each year.

28. **Which populations are at most risk for TB?**

The disease is most prevalent in urban areas. Several populations have been identified as having a high incidence of TB:
- Prison inmates
- Alcoholics
- Drug-dependent persons
- Homeless persons
- Persons infected with human immunodeficiency virus (HIV)
- Persons in residential care facilities

29. How is TB transmitted?

Infection occurs primarily by inhalation of respiratory droplets aerosolized by coughing, sneezing, or talking. Initial infection usually occurs in the lower lung fields because there is greater distribution of ventilation to the lung bases. Bacterial multiplication proceeds slowly, both in the initial focus and in metastatic foci. Approximately 6 to 8 weeks after initial infection, specific cell-mediated immunity develops, providing effective killing of most organisms and containment of infection by the formation of granulomas. The TB skin test becomes positive at this time. Reactivation infection occurs in about 10% of infected patients. Reactivation occurs within 2 years after initial infection. When reactivation occurs, it most commonly is situated in the apical posterior segment of the upper lobes of the lungs, which is rarely the site of primary infection. Primary infection is usually asymptomatic.

30. What are the common manifestations associated with TB?

- Anorexia
- Weight loss
- Fever
- Night sweats
- Hemoptysis

31. How is TB treated?

Multiple drugs should be used to prevent the emergence of drug-resistant organisms. If treatment fails, drugs need to be changed in combination rather than singularly. Single daily drug doses are preferred. Repeat sputum cultures for acid-fast bacilli (AFB). No matter what regimen is chosen, it is important to follow up patients closely to ensure compliance and to monitor drug effectiveness and toxicity. Monthly liver functions studies should be done because hepatic toxicity is associated with some of the medications.

32. Describe the chest radiograph findings associated with pleural effusion.

The chest radiograph is the major diagnostic test used to identify a pleural effusion. A posteroanterior (PA) and lateral view generally identifies an effusion. With as little as 100 mL of pleural fluid, a blunting of the costophrenic angle can be seen on the lateral chest radiograph. Blunting is seen on the PA view with ≥200 mL of pleural fluid. Identification of the underlying cause of the effusion is also necessary for treatment to be effective.

33. What is the role of thoracentesis in the management of pleural effusion?

A thoracentesis relieves symptoms by draining fluid from the pleural space. The patient should be placed in an upright position while sitting on the edge of the bed, preferably with his or her arms resting on a table. The fluid should be removed slowly, with no more than 1000 to 1500 mL removed at a time. If the patient complains of chest pain or begins to cough, the procedure should be stopped. Additionally, the fluid obtained should be sent for laboratory examination. The presence of protein, lactate dehydrogenase, red cells, or white cells would indicate that the effusion is an exudate. If the fluid appears cloudy, blood tinged, or has pus in it, a Gram stain should be done. A repeat chest radiograph is done after the procedure to ensure that a pneumothorax has not developed and to assess the effectiveness of the thoracentesis.

34. What is a pulmonary embolus (PE)?

A PE occurs when a venous thrombus lodges in the vasculature of one of the lungs. A PE is not seen as an independent disease but is associated with another disease process.

35. What are the causes of PE?

A PE can also occur as a result of other fluids or material that enter the vasculature. Deep vein thrombus, amniotic fluid during pregnancy, fat embolus, air, and iatrogenic causes are all sources for a PE.

36. Which patients are at risk for a PE from a deep vein thrombus (DVT)?

Three factors contribute to a patient's risk for developing DVT and thus a PE. Venous stasis as associated with prolonged bedrest, hypercoagulability as seen in patients with disseminated intravascular coagulation, and vascular injury from trauma or surgery are referred to as Virchow's triad and can help to identify patients at risk for the development of a DVT.

37. What is the best therapy for treating a PE?

The best treatment for a PE is *prevention*. Identification of the patients at risk and implementation of therapies directed at prevention of a DVT will do the most to prevent a PE from occurring. Early ambulation after surgery, the use of intermittent compression devices, and the use of prophylactic heparin or warfarin are common effective therapies.

38. What are the manifestations of a PE?

The classic manifestations of a PE are rarely seen, because only a small percentage of patients present with these complaints. The manifestations may include the following:
- Dyspnea
- Pleuritic chest pain
- Hemoptysis
- Cough
- Splinting of the ribs with breathing

- Dyspnea
- Tachycardia
- Hypotension
- Near-syncope
- Apprehension

39. **What diagnostic studies are used to identify a PE?**

A chest radiograph, ventilation/perfusion ($\dot{V}/\dot{Q}$) scan of the lungs, CT scan, and arterial blood gas study are useful in the diagnosis of a PE. The gold standard is a pulmonary angiogram.
- Chest radiograph is used to primarily exclude any other causes of the patient's symptoms such as a pneumothorax.
- $\dot{V}/\dot{Q}$ scan is a nuclear medicine study that compares ventilation defects in the lungs with perfusion (vascular) defects. In the case of a pulmonary embolus, ventilation is usually normal but there is a defect in perfusion. If the $\dot{V}/\dot{Q}$ scan is negative, then a PE is ruled out. If the scan shows a low to high probability of a PE, then further testing is required to confirm a PE.
- CT scan is capable of detecting defective filling in the segmental or larger pulmonary arteries but not in subsegmental arteries. Positive CT scan results in association with other manifestations can help confirm the diagnosis of PE. A negative CT scan does not rule out a PE, especially if other clinical manifestations support its presence. Spiral CT scan is also being used.
- Arterial blood gas results show respiratory alkalosis and hypoxemia. However, the absence of hypoxemia does not rule out a PE.

40. **Describe the treatment of PE.**

A PE is treated emergently. Treatment focuses on emergent relief of symptoms and identification of the underlying source of the PE. Anticoagulation should be started immediately. Typically, an infusion of heparin is started. The purpose of this infusion is not to dissolve the clot but to prevent further thrombosis (inhibit growth of the PE). This allows the fibrinolytic system to proceed with the process of naturally dissolving the embolus. Low-molecular-weight dextran may be used as an alternative clot preventing medication. For long-term anticoagulation, warfarin, aspirin, or other antiplatelet drugs are used.

41. **What is the role of thrombolytic therapy in the treatment of PE?**

Thrombolytic therapy such as streptokinase, tissue plasminogen activator (TPA), or urokinase is typically used in the management of a PE that is causing hemodynamic instability or severe respiratory compromise.

42. **What is pulmonary hypertension?**

Pulmonary hypertension exists when the pressure in the pulmonary vascular bed is consistently elevated above a mean pressure of 30 mm Hg.

43. **What risk factors are associated with pulmonary hypertension?**

Pulmonary hypertension usually occurs secondary to a pre-existing illness. Patients at risk for developing secondary pulmonary hypertension are those with intracardiac shunting, cardiomyopathy, emphysema, scleroderma, lupus erythematosus, PE, sickle cell disease, or sleep apnea. When an underlying cause for the pulmonary hypertension cannot be identified, it is referred to as idiopathic or primary pulmonary hypertension (PPH).

44. **What early manifestations are associated with pulmonary hypertension?**

Typically a patient with pulmonary hypertension has very few symptoms until the disease is well advanced. The pulmonary vasculature is able to accommodate large increases in pulmonary blood flow before the patient or health care provider notices symptoms. Fatigue and dyspnea on exertion are usually the complaints that bring a patient to seek medical attention. These general symptoms can frequently be attributed to anxiety, overwork, or being physically unfit. If left untreated, there is a 45% to 50% mortality rate at 2 to 3 years after the onset of symptoms.

45. **What are the later manifestations associated with pulmonary hypertension?**

As the disease progresses, the patient may present with chest pain, syncope or presyncope, hemoptysis, hoarseness, and symptoms of right-sided heart failure such as peripheral edema, the development of third or fourth heart sounds, and arterial hypoxemia that does not respond well to oxygen supplement.

46. **What is the definitive diagnostic test in the evaluation of pulmonary hypertension?**

The only definitive test for pulmonary hypertension is a right heart catheterization.

47. **What other diagnostic testing may be used?**

- Pulmonary function test
- Echocardiogram
- Chest radiograph
- CT scan

48. **Describe the treatment of pulmonary hypertension.**

Treatment of pulmonary hypertension includes the use of supplemental oxygen. This helps control the patient's hypoxia and reduce afterload on the right ventricle. Anticoagulation is necessary to prevent the development of venous thrombus and pulmonary embolism. Vasodilator therapy is also used in the treatment of pulmonary hypertension. This therapy is not very effective in patients with secondary pulmonary hypertension. Oral medications (calcium channel blockers) such as nifedipine and diltiazem are typically used. In patients with PPH, epoprostenol (Flolan), a potent intravenous (IV) vasodilator, can be used. Lung transplantation can occasionally be used as a treatment for pulmonary hypertension when all other therapies have been exhausted.

49. What is epoprostenol (Flolan) and what is the mechanism of action?

Flolan is a prostacyclin used in the treatment of PPH. Flolan mimics the effects of naturally occurring prostacyclin but has a very short half-life of 3 to 5 minutes and therefore must be administered in a continuous IV form via a central line. Initiation of the medication is done in the cardiac catheterization lab or intensive care unit and titration of the dose is done slowly over several weeks to months.

50. What are the common side effects and problems associated with the use of epoprostenol (Flolan)?

The most common complaints from patients on Flolan occur with the initiation of therapy and with dose increases. Jaw pain, facial flushing, diarrhea, and headaches are the most common complaints. These symptoms generally resolve within a few days of the dose adjustment. Line infection and breakage are long-term problems frequently seen in patients on Flolan therapy. Frequent or prolonged manipulation of the catheter and site can result in line sepsis or breakage and the need to replace the catheter. The drug is unstable and once mixed with diluent must be kept refrigerated. While being infused, the drug must be stored on ice packs.

51. What are the desired results of Flolan therapy?

Ideally, a decrease in the patient's pulmonary pressures should be seen with an increase in the Flolan dose. Frequently, the reduction in these pressures is not as significant as might be expected, although the patient's 6-minute walk test, pulmonary vascular resistance, and cardiac output are improved. It has been suggested that chronic use of Flolan also has nonvasodilating effects such as inotropy and vascular remodeling.

52. What other pharmacological alternatives are available to the patient with pulmonary hypertension?

Tracleer (bosentan) is a recently approved oral agent for the treatment of pulmonary hypertension. Tracleer blocks the action of endothelin, a naturally occurring substance in the body that causes narrowing of blood vessels and thus elevation in pulmonary pressures. Tracleer can be used in patients with mild PPH and in patients with secondary pulmonary hypertension. The two major risks when using this medication are the risk of liver toxicity and the drug's potential damage to a fetus. The drug is started at a half dose of 62.5 mg twice daily and increased to 125 mg twice daily after the first month if liver enzyme elevation is not present. The primary tools used to assess the effectiveness of

Tracleer are the 6-minute walk test, CT scan, monitoring of liver enzymes, and the patient's subjective reporting. Tracleer is only slightly less expensive than Flolan but does not have the risks of a continuous infusion associated with it.

Remodulin is a synthetic form of prostacyclin that can be delivered subcutaneously. It is a more stable form of prostacyclin than Flolan with a half-life of 4 to 6 hours. It is delivered via an infusion pump through a subcutaneous needle, usually inserted in the abdomen. The side effects of Remodulin are similar to those of Flolan—headache, diarrhea, jaw pain, and flushing—but the patient may also complain of pain at the needle insertion site. The risk of line infection and sepsis seen with Flolan is less with Remodulin.

Beraprost and *iloprost* are oral and inhaled forms, respectively, of prostacyclins currently being investigated.

53. What is a primary pneumothorax?

A primary pneumothorax is also referred to as a *simple pneumothorax*. A primary pneumothorax occurs abruptly as a result of the rupture of a bleb or cyst in the apical lung region.

54. How does a pneumothorax occur?

A pneumothorax occurs when air enters the normally gas-free pleural space. The pleural space is located between the visceral pleura and the parietal pleura. Normally this space contains a small amount of pleural fluid (5 to 15 mL). The pleural fluid serves as a lubricant between the two pleurae. Pleural pressure is normally slightly negative compared with atmospheric pressure. When the pleural space is penetrated, it is exposed to positive atmospheric pressure. This causes the lung to collapse inward. The underlying cause of the pneumothorax determines the severity of the pneumothorax, the symptoms, and the treatment.

55. Describe the typical patient in whom a primary pneumothorax develops.

The typical patient is a young man 20 to 35 years of age. The patient is usually tall and slender in build and in good health. About 30% of these patients have a recurrence within 3 years.

56. What are the common clinical manifestations associated with a primary pneumothorax?

The clinical manifestations of a primary pneumothorax are directly related to the size of the pneumothorax. A small pneumothorax that raises the intrapleural pressure only slightly causes few symptoms and is well tolerated by an otherwise healthy patient. With a larger pneumothorax, the patient typically complains of sudden-onset pain that is pleuritic in nature. This pain lessens as air accumulates in the pleural space and separation of the pleural lining is complete.

Eventually, the character of the pain becomes a chronic dull ache. The patient becomes tachycardic and short of breath. Auscultation of breath sounds reveals diminished or absent breath sounds on the affected side.

57. What electrocardiographic (ECG) findings are associated with pneumothorax?

An ECG may show signs that can be misinterpreted as a subendocardial myocardial infarction: decreased voltage, axis shifts, and T wave inversion across the pericardium.

58. How is the diagnosis of primary pneumothorax made?

The diagnosis of primary pneumothorax is made from the patient's history, physical examination, and radiographic studies. The chest radiograph shows a partially collapsed lung outlined by the visceral pleural line. An end-expiratory chest film or a decubitus film may be needed to help visualize a small pneumothorax.

59. How is a pneumothorax treated?

If the pneumothorax is small (<20%) and the patient is asymptomatic, the patient does not require any treatment other than observation. The pneumothorax will reabsorb within 1 to 2 weeks. Intervention is required for a pneumothorax greater than 20%. A chest tube is inserted and connected to a water seal and suction. A chest radiograph should be obtained to confirm correct placement of the chest tube. The chest tube is left in place until evidence of an air leak is absent for at least 24 hours and the lung appears re-expanded on chest film. In patients in whom this therapy is not effective or who have recurrence of the pneumothorax, additional surgical interventions may be required.

60. Describe other options in the treatment of pneumothorax.

The goal of an invasive surgical intervention is to irritate the pleural tissue and cause the development of adhesions and scar tissue, thus preventing a future recurrence of a pneumothorax. One option is to introduce a sclerosing agent (doxycycline or talc) into the pleural space via the chest tube. This is a painful procedure. Another alternative is to perform thoracoscopic examination of the lung and pleura. General anesthesia is required for this procedure but it allows direct examination of the chest for air leaks, blebs, and repair. Pleurodesis can also be done via a thoracoscopic procedure. Pleurodesis is the mechanical irritation of the pleura such that scar tissue develops, preventing a future pneumothorax. Chemicals, talc, and pleural abrasion are examples of ways to mechanically stimulate the development of scar tissue.

61. What is a secondary or complicated spontaneous pneumothorax?

A secondary pneumothorax occurs in patients with underlying pulmonary disease. Some diseases in which a pneumothorax can be seen include COPD, interstitial fibrosis, neoplasm, infection, and *Pneumocystis carinii* pneumonia.

62. **Describe the difference in managing a primary versus a secondary pneumothorax.**

The diagnosis is made using the same set of criteria as previously described and treatment is similar. The major difference between the two types of pneumothorax is that a patient with a secondary pneumothorax, because of the underlying disease, must be identified and treated quickly. These patients tend to have less pulmonary and cardiac reserve and the situation can rapidly deteriorate to become life threatening. In patients who are being mechanically ventilated, adjustment of the ventilator to a high-frequency, low-pressure ventilator may be necessary to manage the air leak and prevent further exacerbation.

63. **Describe additional causes of pneumothorax.**

- Either penetrating or nonpenetrating trauma to the chest is another cause of pneumothorax. Typical sources for this type of pneumothorax are rib fractures, stab or bullet wounds, and deceleration injury to the chest, such as occurs in an automobile accident.
- An iatrogenic pneumothorax is seen as a complication associated with subclavian line placement, thoracentesis, or transbronchial lung biopsy.
- A catamenial pneumothorax can occur in women with endometriosis. It typically occurs on the right side of the chest in women younger than 30 years of age. A spontaneous pneumothorax occurs within 48 hours of the start of menstruation and is attributed to minute endometrial implants on the surface of the lung. Treatment includes ovulation-suppressing drugs and chemical pleurodesis.

64. **What physiological changes occur in a patient with tension pneumothorax?**

In a tension pneumothorax, air is allowed to continuously enter the pleural space. This causes an accumulation of positive pressure within the pleural space and significant lung collapse. If extreme, there can be shifting of the trachea and mediastinum to the contralateral side and even collapse of the uninvolved lung. The patient exhibits hypotension and hemodynamic instability. This situation is a medical emergency and requires immediate intervention with a chest tube. If the patient is being mechanically ventilated at the time of the tension pneumothorax, the situation is even more urgent. Mechanical ventilation only increases the positive pressure within the pleural space and exacerbates the patient's symptoms.

65. **How is asthma characterized?**

- Airway inflammation
- Airway hyperresponsiveness
- Airflow obstruction that is variable

66. **What are the clinical manifestations associated with exacerbation of asthma?**

- Dyspnea
- Cough
- Audible wheezing

- Chest tightness
- Tachypnea
- Use of accessory muscles
- Diaphoresis
- Difficulty in speaking and completing sentences

67. How is asthma diagnosed?

- Clinical history
- Reversible airway obstruction by pulmonary function testing

68. Which disease entities should be considered in the differential diagnosis of asthma?

- Chronic bronchitis
- Upper airway obstruction
- Vocal cord dysfunction
- Heart failure
- Pulmonary embolism
- Aspiration

69. What are some of the complications that may be associated with an acute exacerbation of asthma?

- Barotrauma
- Respiratory failure
- Cardiac dysrhythmias
- Lobar lung collapse
- Death

70. What is the mainstay of treatment for patients with asthma?

- Beta receptor agonists
- Corticosteroids (oral and inhaled)
- Control of environmental allergens

🔑 Key Points

- COPD is more prevalent in men and increases with advancing age.
- The best treatment for pulmonary embolus is prevention.
- Medication noncompliance is the most common reason for the development of multidrug-resistant TB.
- The natural progression of COPD is correlated with FEV_1.
- Patients with pulmonary hypertension usually are asymptomatic until the disease is advanced.
- Patients with pneumothorax may have electrocardiogram changes.

Internet Resources

The Lung Association: Asthma:
www.lung.ca/asthma

American Academy of Allergy, Asthma, and Immunology:
www.aaaai.org

Global Initiative for Chronic Obstructive Lung Disease:
www.goldcopd.com

The Lung Association: Chronic Lung Disease:
www.lung.ca/copd

EMedicine: Pneumonia, Bacterial:
www.emedicine.com/EMERG/topic465.htm

Bibliography

Bordow, R.A., Ries, A.L., & Morris, T.A. (Eds.). (2001). *Manual of clinical problems in pulmonary medicine* (5th ed.). Philadelphia: Lippincott Williams & Wilkins.

Fishman, A.P. (Ed.). (1994). *Pulmonary diseases and disorders companion handbook* (2nd ed.). New York: McGraw-Hill.

Hayes, D.D. (2001). Stemming the tide of pleural effusion. *Nursing2001, 31,* 5, 49-52.

Hayes, G.B. (1998). *Pulmonary hypertension—A patient's survival guide.* Silver Spring, MD: Pulmonary Hypertension Association.

Rubin, L.J., et al. (2002). Bosentan therapy for pulmonary arterial hypertension. *The New England Journal of Medicine, 346,* 896-903.

Ziesche, R., et al. (1999). A preliminary study of long-term treatment with interferon gamma–1b and low-dose prednisolone in patients with idiopathic pulmonary fibrosis. *The New England Journal of Medicine, 341,* 1264-1269.

Cardiac Disorders

Virginia Buckley-Blaskovich and Carol Twomey

1. **What are the most common causes of aortic stenosis?**
   - Rheumatic disease
   - Calcification
   - Congenital abnormality (bicuspid valve)

2. **What is the clinical significance of a bicuspid aortic valve?**

   A bicuspid aortic valve has no significance until it begins to deteriorate. If the valve functions normally, then the valve does not need to be replaced. There is a 3% risk of penetrance to the offspring in those people found to have a bicuspid aortic valve.

3. **What is the normal aortic valve area?**

   The normal aortic valve area is 2.5 to 3.5 cm^2.

4. **What is considered critical aortic stenosis?**

   An aortic valve area ≤ 0.7 cm^2 is considered critical aortic stenosis.

5. **What are the classic symptoms of aortic stenosis?**
   - Syncope
   - Angina
   - Dyspnea (heart failure)

6. **How is aortic stenosis diagnosed?**

   The murmur associated with aortic stenosis is described as a systolic crescendo-decrescendo murmur auscultated at the second right intercostal space and along the left sternal border, radiating to the carotids bilaterally. Other physical examination findings may include an atrial gallop, a displaced apical impulse, left ventricular heaves, and decreased carotid upstroke. These findings would prompt an echocardiogram to confirm the presence of the stenotic lesion. Aortic stenosis can also be detected with cardiac catheterization.

7. **What are treatment options for patients with moderate to critical aortic stenosis?**

   - Monitor for progression of symptoms
   - Serial echocardiograms
   - Endocarditis prophylaxis
   - Surgical intervention if symptomatic and valve area less than 1.0 cm^2

8. **What valvular choices are available when aortic valve replacement surgery is indicated?**

   The standard recommendations for aortic valve replacement are (1) the pericardial aortic valve for patients 70 years of age or older or for patients with contraindications to taking blood thinners and (2) the mechanical valve for patients younger than 70 years of age or for patients who are already on blood thinners. The limiting factor of pericardial valves is its lack of longevity. New technologies are being clinically investigated to increase the pericardial valve longevity as well as to decrease the gradient over the valve prosthesis. New pericardial aortic root replacements have low valvular gradients with an approximate longevity of 15 to 20 years. Homografts remain the best valvular choice in the treatment of endocarditis. Mechanical valve replacements have greater longevity, but they require long-term anticoagulation with warfarin. These valves have low valvular gradients and are effective in both the mitral and aortic positions.

9. **What is the difference between an aortic dissection and an aortic aneurysm?**

   An aortic aneurysm is an outpouching of the aortic wall, which is caused by high blood pressure, smoking, a family history, or a congenital connective tissue disorder. There are two types of aneurysms: fusiform and saccular. Fusiform aneurysms are the most common. They are long and wide, whereas a saccular aneurysm is a round outpouching of the aortic wall. Aortic aneurysms have an intact intimal layer.

   Aortic dissection is the abrupt development of a tear between the intimal and medial layers of the aorta, through which a column of blood is driven by the force of the arterial pressure into the aortic wall, thereby creating a second channel of blood flow. Aortic dissections are classified as either type A or type B using the Stanford classification system. *Type A* aortic dissections are usually emergent because the tear begins in the ascending aorta and can extend distally through the aortic arch and descending thoracic aorta. The tear can also extend proximally to the aortic valve. *Type B* aortic dissections have a tear site just distal to the left subclavian artery and can extend into the descending thoracic and abdominal aorta.

10. **What are the most common causes of aortic aneurysms?**

   - Uncontrolled hypertension
   - Smoking
   - Congenital abnormality such as bicuspid aortic valve or coarctation of the aorta

- Connective tissue disorders such as Marfan's syndrome and Ehlers-Danlos syndrome
- Family history

11. What is the preferred treatment method for both type A and type B aortic dissections?

The treatment method for acute *type A* aortic dissections is emergent surgery. This surgery includes replacement of the ascending aorta with a hemiarch repair. Usually the aortic valve can be repaired or resuspended. If the type A dissection tear destroys the aortic valve, then sometimes the aortic valve must be replaced. Once surgery has been performed, the continued treatment plan includes aggressive hypertension control. This helps decrease the risk of aneurysmal formation of the residual dissection that extends into the descending thoracic aorta.

The method of treatment for an acute or chronic *type B* dissection is aggressive hypertension control. Initially this might require hospitalization for intravenous hypertension medication in order to tightly control the blood pressure. An optimal blood pressure for an acute type B aortic dissection is systolic pressure less than 135 mm Hg. Surgery in an acute type B dissection is only indicated when there is a malperfusion syndrome or an aortic rupture. Surgical intervention for acute type B dissection has a 50% rate for mortality and morbidity, including paralysis. Long-term serial computed tomography (CT) scanning in both type A and type B dissections is necessary to ensure the surgical repair is intact and no pseudoaneurysms have formed. The residual dissection must be monitored to ensure there is no aneurysmal formation of the dissected aorta.

12. What is the first line of pharmacological therapy used in aortic aneurysms and dissections?

The first-line agent used in aortic dissections as well as aortic aneurysms is beta-blocker therapy. These agents have been shown in the Marfan's population to be effective in decreasing the growth rate of the aorta. This concept has been extrapolated to the larger population. Beta blockers decrease the dP/dt (diastolic pressure/diastolic time) ratio or the stress on the aortic wall, thereby decreasing the risk of aneurysmal growth. Beta-blocker therapy only reduces the aortic wall stress. Hypertension management also needs to be implemented. If beta blockers alone do not maintain the goal blood pressure, then other antihypertensive agents should be used in combination with the beta blockers. A contraindication to beta-blocker therapy is significant chronic obstructive pulmonary disease (COPD) or aortic insufficiency.

13. What is mitral valve prolapse (MVP)?

MVP is a genetic connective tissue disorder that primarily affects the mitral leaflets, chordae tendinea, and annulus and that may progress to clinically significant mitral regurgitation.

14. **What are the common symptoms associated with MVP?**
    - Chest pain
    - Dizziness
    - Dyspnea
    - Fatigue
    - Exercise intolerance

    The patient may be asymptomatic.

15. **What is the hallmark auscultatory finding associated with MVP?**
    - Mid-systolic click, which varies with left ventricular volume
    - Late systolic murmur

16. **What are potential complications that may occur in patients with MVP?**
    - Dysrhythmias
    - Sudden death
    - Endocarditis
    - Embolic events
    - Mitral regurgitation

17. **What is mitral valvular regurgitation?**

    Mitral regurgitation occurs when the mitral valve becomes incompetent either by defective function of the leaflets, papillary muscle, chordae tendinea, or enlargement of the orifice.

18. **What are the most common causes of mitral regurgitation?**
    - Rheumatic disease
    - MVP
    - Myxomatous degeneration
    - Ischemic heart disease

19. **When should mitral valvular regurgitation be surgically corrected?**

    Mitral regurgitation should be surgically corrected when the ejection fraction begins to fall or the left ventricular end-diastolic size increases, or when the patient develops manifestations of heart failure such as dyspnea, fatigue, or atrial fibrillation.

    Reconstruction of the mitral valve is preferred over replacement. Complex reconstruction of the leaflets and placing a ring over the orifice is initially the correction preferred.

20. **What happens to left ventricular function after surgical intervention on the mitral valve?**

When mitral regurgitation is corrected, the ejection fraction generally is lowered. Once the regurgitation of the valve has been corrected, the loss of the low impedance pathway for blood flow retrograde across the mitral valve may increase left ventricular afterload, thus unmasking pre-existing ventricular dysfunction.

21. **What surgical options are available in patients with mitral valve disease?**

Correction of atrial fibrillation after mitral valve repair is also helpful in maintaining good left ventricular function. Additional surgical procedures such as radiofrequency ablation may be performed to aid in the control or elimination of atrial fibrillation after mitral valve repair.

There are also experimental devices that "girdle" the ventricle and do not allow it to dilate after the mitral regurgitation (MR) is corrected. The procedure consists of removed ventricular tissue between the heads of the papillary muscle posteriorly when repairing the MV. It was thought that by removing this tissue, the ventricle would not *continue* to dilate. This procedure is controversial today, however, and has fallen out of favor.

The *ACORN/CORCAP* device is an experimental procedure that girdles the ventricle. It is a caplike device that is placed over the ventricle during MV surgery. It is hypothesized that the device will not allow the ventricle to dilate after MV surgery. Why the ventricle continues to dilate in idiopathic disease is unknown, so it is also not known whether the girdling device will prevent ventricle dilation over time.

22. **What is an atrial myxoma?**

Myxomas are the most common cardiac tumors. The tumors most frequently arise from the left atrium (75%) as compared to the right atrium (25%).

Myxomas may present at any age, but they are more common in the fourth decade. Most are found in women. Most myxomas are incidental findings associated with cardiac catheterization or echocardiograms done for the patient.

23. **How are atrial myxomas diagnosed?**

Myxomas are not usually diagnosed clinically. However symptoms may include dyspnea that is improved with lying down, as well as the manifestation of heart failure including mitral regurgitation, mitral stenosis, or both. These symptoms occur mainly because the myxoma occludes either the mitral valve or pulmonary vein. This accounts for the symptoms abating with position change as the tumor moves out of position of interfering with atrial outflow across the mitral or tricuspid valve.

24. What is the state-of-the-art medical therapy for heart failure (HF)?

The mainstay of HF therapy consists of drug therapy that affects the neuro-hormonal effects of HF on the body. These include angiotensin-converting enzyme (ACE) inhibitors, beta blockers, cardiac glycosides, diuretics, and anticoagulants. Patient teaching is also an important mainstay in the treatment of HF.

- Since the mid-1980s, *ACE inhibitors* have been used to control the angiotensin-renin system in the kidney. Activation of this system is triggered by low cardiac output. It causes the kidneys to secrete renin, which causes vasoconstriction. This vasoconstriction, as well as the resultant elevation of the systemic vascular resistance, affects the ability of the left ventricle to empty. Cardiac output is then affected.
- *Beta blockers* have been used since the mid-1990s to deactivate the effect of the sympathetic nervous system in HF. These effects include tachycardia and increased afterload. They must be added cautiously and are not given to patients who present with acute heart failure or pulmonary edema.
- The use of *digoxin* in patients with heart failure is generally accepted.
- *Diuretics* tailored to fit the patient's needs are also used. Generally patients are asked to weigh themselves every day, and they can increase or decrease their diuretics in response to their weight.
- Most patients with ejection fraction less than 20% are also placed on *warfarin (Coumadin)*.
- Extensive *teaching* in fluid and diet control is also often overlooked but is a very important aspect of good heart failure management.

25. What are the indications for cardiac transplantation?

In general, patients are referred for cardiac transplantation after they have failed traditional medical therapy for heart failure. This therapy consists of ACE inhibitors or angiotensin-blocking agents, beta blockers, diuretics, anti-coagulants, and in most cases digoxin.

Despite optimal medical therapy, patients may eventually become tolerant to the therapy or the disease process itself may progress. At this point, some patients are referred to a transplant center for cardiac transplantation.

26. What is pericarditis?

Pericarditis is an inflammation of the pericardium.

27. What are the possible etiologies of pericarditis?

- Postcardiac surgery
- Post myocardial infarction (MI)
- Viral infection

- Renal disease
- Lupus erythematosus
- Scleroderma
- Rheumatoid arthritis
- Rheumatic fever
- Cancer

28. What are the common symptoms associated with pericarditis?

- Chest pain especially with inspiration
- Low-grade fever, chills
- Shortness of breath
- Cough

29. How is pericarditis diagnosed?

Pericarditis can be diagnosed through electrocardiographic (ECG) changes with ST segment elevation with no Q waves to suggest infarction. Dysrhythmias are not uncommon including the potential for atrial fibrillation. An echocardiogram is often useful in the diagnosis, because it can detect the presence of a pericardial effusion. If the pericarditis is not the result of recent cardiac surgery, a sedimentation rate may be helpful. Chronic or recurrent pericarditis may require a CT scan or magnetic resonance imaging to evaluate the thickening of the pericardium.

30. What is the treatment for pericarditis?

Currently pericarditis is treated with nonsteroidal anti-inflammatory drug (NSAID) therapy. The NSAID therapy (e.g., ibuprofen or Indocin) helps decrease the inflammatory process. If the pericarditis is not resolved with the administration of the NSAID therapy, then steroids are prescribed for a short course of 2 weeks. Colchicine, a gout medication, has been shown to be of benefit in the treatment of acute pericarditis.

31. What is the most common dysrhythmia after cardiac surgery?

The most common dysrhythmia after cardiac surgery is atrial fibrillation.

32. What is the most common treatment for atrial fibrillation after cardiac surgery?

Preoperative and postoperative beta blockade is useful in preventing atrial fibrillation. It has also been recommended in high-risk patients that amiodarone, either intravenous or oral, be used both before and after surgery to prevent atrial fibrillation. If amiodarone is used, it is short term due to the potential side effects associated with long-term use.

33. When is coronary artery bypass grafting indicated?

The clinical and anatomical indications for coronary artery bypass grafting include the following:
* Left main stenosis greater than 50%
* Three-vessel coronary disease with an impaired left ventricular function
* Two-vessel disease with significant proximal left anterior descending (LAD) stenosis
* Severely depressed left ventricular function with evidence for reversible ischemia
* Left main equivalent with significant (>70%) stenosis of the proximal LAD and proximal left circumflex artery
* Disabling angina despite maximal medical therapy
* Ongoing ischemia/infarction not responsive to maximal nonsurgical therapy
* Life-threatening ventricular dysrhythmias

34. What is off-pump coronary artery bypass grafting?

Off-pump coronary artery bypass grafting is bypass surgery without the use of the cardiopulmonary bypass machine. It is performed on the slow beating heart with a special cardiac stabilizer. Its interest comes from the belief that the cardiopulmonary bypass machine is associated with many of the postoperative complications including neurocognitive impairments.

35. What are the perceived advantages of off-pump coronary artery bypass surgery?

* Neurocognitive preservation
* Cost reduction
* Decreased hospital cost
* Decreased inflammatory response
* Decreased volume overload

36. What is the perceived disadvantage of the off-pump coronary artery bypass procedure?

The perceived disadvantage of the off-pump coronary artery bypass procedure is decreased bypass graft patency.

37. What are the recommendations for myocardial revascularization?

Myocardial revascularization is recommended to achieve the following goals:
* Alleviation of symptoms of myocardial ischemia
* Decrease the risk of mortality and morbidity
* Treat or prevent complications of coronary ischemia such as myocardial infarction, dysrhythmias, and heart failure

38. What conduits can be used to perform coronary artery bypass grafting?

Coronary Artery Bypass Grafting Conduits

Type of Conduits	Patency Rate	Duration of Patency
Left internal mammary artery/right internal mammary artery graft	83%	10 years
Saphenous vein graft	74%	5 years
	41%	10 years
Radial artery	85%	5 years

39. What treatment alternatives are available for patients who are not candidates for coronary artery bypass grafting?

If a patient is not a coronary artery bypass candidate, then optimization of his or her medical management is always the first choice. If the patient remains symptomatic despite medical therapy, then there are several other treatment options. The first is a noninvasive approach called *enhanced external counter pulsation,* or EECP. This treatment is used to relieve the symptoms of angina and shortness of breath by stimulating or increasing coronary blood flow and collateralization. The next two are surgical options. The first is a procedure called *transmyocardial revascularization.* This, too, is performed to increase coronary artery blood flow by stimulating angiogenesis or coronary collateralization. The third option is a *cardiac transplant* for ischemic cardiomyopathy.

40. What are the evidence-based national treatment recommendations for hyperlipidemia?

The recommendations for the treatment of hyperlipidemia according to the evidence-based standard are published by the National Guidelines Clearinghouse of the Agency for Healthcare Research and Quality (Adult Treatment Panel III, 2001). (See also the figure on pp. 98 and 99.)

Pharmacological therapy can be used in conjunction with nonpharmacological therapy such as dietary therapy, weight reduction and physical activity. Pharmacological treatment should be initiated after lifestyle modifications have been unsuccessful after a 12-week trial.

- Patients *without coronary heart disease* and with *fewer than two risk factors* should be considered for drug therapy when the low-density lipoprotein (LDL) is more than 190 mg/dL or higher with the goal of therapy to have an LDL less than 160 mg/dL.
- Patients *without coronary heart disease* and with *two or more risk factors* should be considered for drug therapy when the LDL is greater than 160 mg/dL or higher with the goal of therapy to have an LDL less than 130 mg/dL.

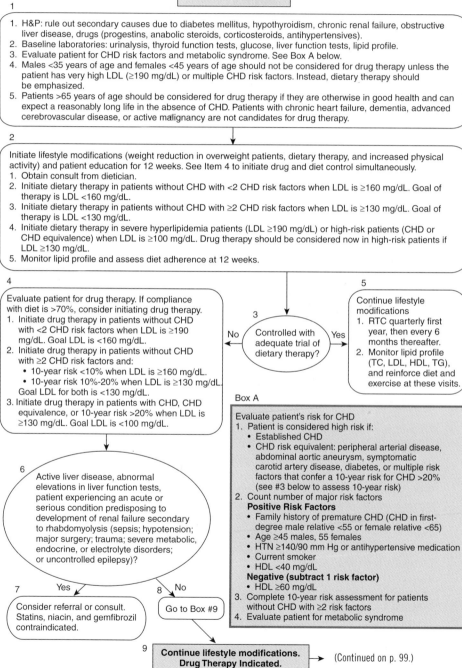

Hyperlipidemia. (From Hyperlipidemia. (2002). Huntsville, TX: University of Texas Medical Branch Correctional Managed Care.)

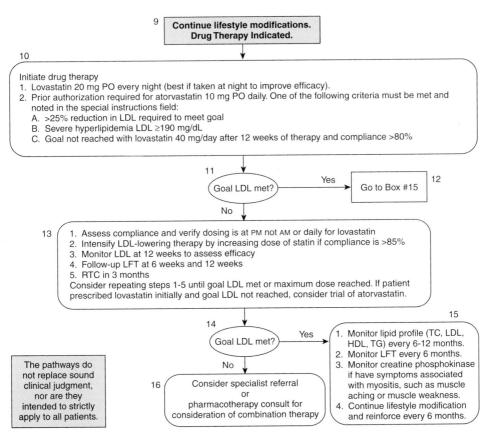

9 | **Continue lifestyle modifications. Drug Therapy Indicated.**

10
Initiate drug therapy
1. Lovastatin 20 mg PO every night (best if taken at night to improve efficacy).
2. Prior authorization required for atorvastatin 10 mg PO daily. One of the following criteria must be met and noted in the special instructions field:
   A. >25% reduction in LDL required to meet goal
   B. Severe hyperlipidemia LDL ≥190 mg/dL
   C. Goal not reached with lovastatin 40 mg/day after 12 weeks of therapy and compliance >80%

11
Goal LDL met? — Yes → 12 Go to Box #15

No

13
1. Assess compliance and verify dosing is at PM not AM or daily for lovastatin
2. Intensify LDL-lowering therapy by increasing dose of statin if compliance is >85%
3. Monitor LDL at 12 weeks to assess efficacy
4. Follow-up LFT at 6 weeks and 12 weeks
5. RTC in 3 months
Consider repeating steps 1-5 until goal LDL met or maximum dose reached. If patient prescribed lovastatin initially and goal LDL not reached, consider trial of atorvastatin.

14
Goal LDL met? — Yes →

No

15
1. Monitor lipid profile (TC, LDL, HDL, TG) every 6-12 months.
2. Monitor LFT every 6 months.
3. Monitor creatine phosphokinase if have symptoms associated with myositis, such as muscle aching or muscle weakness.
4. Continue lifestyle modification and reinforce every 6 months.

16
Consider specialist referral
or
pharmacotherapy consult for consideration of combination therapy

The pathways do not replace sound clinical judgment, nor are they intended to strictly apply to all patients.

Hyperlipidemia (cont'd from p. 98). (From Hyperlipidemia. (2002). Huntsville, TX: University of Texas Medical Branch Correctional Managed Care.)

- Patients *with coronary heart disease* should be considered for drug therapy when the LDL is greater than 130 mg/dL or higher. The goal of therapy for this group of patients is an LDL of 100 mg/dL or less.

The table below provides a summary of choices for the patient with hyperlipidemia. Side effects and cost are listed for each group of antihyperlipidemic, which should be considered when initiating therapy for patients (Adult Treatment Panel III, 2001).

Drugs for Hyperlipidemia

Drug Class	Starting Dose	Adverse Reaction	Contraindications
Statins		Myopathy	Absolute: Liver disease
Lovastatin	20 mg daily	Increase liver function	Certain drugs
Atorvastatin	10 mg daily	test values	

Continued

Drugs for Hyperlipidemia—cont'd

Drug Class	Starting Dose	Adverse Reaction	Contraindications
Cholestyramine	4 g four times daily	Gastrointestinal (GI) upset Constipation Decreased absorption of drugs	Absolute: TG >400 mg/dL and dysbetalipoproteinemia Relative: TG >200 mg/dL

Nicotinic acid
    Niacin
 	
    Niacin TR
	
	500 mg three times daily
	500 mg twice daily
		Flushing
		Hyperglycemia
		Hyperuricemia
		GI upset
		Hepatotoxicity
			Absolute: Chronic liver disease, severe gout
			Relative: PUD, diabetes, hyperuricemia

Fibric acid Gemfibrozil	 600 mg twice daily	Dyspepsia Gallstones Myopathy Unexplained non-CHD deaths	Absolute: Severe renal or liver disease

From Hyperlipidemia. (2002). Huntsville, TX: University of Texas Medical Branch Correctional Managed Care. *CHD*, Coronary heart disease; *GI*, gastrointestinal; *PUD*, peptic ulcer disease; *TG*, triglycerides.

41. How is hypertension classified?

The new high blood pressure guidelines were published in the seventh report of the Joint National Committee on High Blood Pressure (JNC VII Report). The classification of hypertension is as follows.

Systolic and Diastolic Blood Pressure

Classification	Blood Pressure Level
Normal	<120/80 mm Hg
Prehypertension	120-139/80-89 mm Hg
Stage I hypertension	140-159/90-99 mm Hg
Stage II hypertension	≥160/100 mm Hg

Data from U.S. Department of Health and Human Services; National Institutes of Health; National Heart, Lung, and Blood Institute. (2003). The Seventh Report of the Joint National Committee on Prevention, Detection, Evaluation, and Treatment of High Blood Pressure. NIH Pub. No. 03-5233. Bethesda, MD: Author.

The new prehypertension classification is to promote awareness and lifestyle modifications such as weight reduction, dietary changes, smoking cessation, and stress reduction.

42. What is the new classification of blood pressure according to the JNC VII Report?

Classification of Blood Pressure

	Systolic Blood Pressure (mm Hg)	Diastolic Blood Pressure (mm Hg)
Normal	<120	<80
Prehypertension	120-139	80-89
Stage I hypertension	140-159	90-99
Stage II hypertension	≥160	≥100

Data from U.S. Department of Health and Human Services; National Institutes of Health; National Heart, Lung, and Blood Institute. (2003). The Seventh Report of the Joint National Committee on Prevention, Detection, Evaluation, and Treatment of High Blood Pressure. NIH Pub. No. 03-5233. Bethesda, MD: Author.

Key Points

- Hypertension management with beta-blocker therapy is the cornerstone of medical management of aortic aneurysm treatment.
- Hypertension should be aggressively treated to prevent long-term complications.
- Patients with mitral valve prolapse are usually asymptomatic.
- The murmur associated with aortic stenosis generally radiates to the carotid arteries.

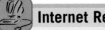

Internet Resources

Heart Center Online:
www.heartcenteronline.com

MDLink Network: Heart Linx—Top Cardiology Articles:
www.mdlinx.com/HeartLinx

American College of Cardiology Foundation: ACC/AHA Guidelines for the Management of Patients with Valvular Heart Disease:
www.acc.org/clinical/guidelines/valvular/dirIndex.htm

Continued

Internet Resources—cont'd

American Heart Association: What Is Coronary Bypass Surgery?:
www.americanheart.org/presenter.jhtml?identifier=3007454

Annals of Thoracic Surgery:
ats.ctsnetjournals.org

Bibliography

ACC/AHA Task Force (1999). ACC/AHA guidelines for coronary artery bypass graft surgery: Executive summary and recommendations. *Circulation, 100,* 1464-1480.

Adult Treatment Panel III. (2001). National Guidelines Clearinghouse of the Agency for Healthcare Research and Quality adapted from Expert Panel on Detection, Evaluation, and Treatment of High Blood Cholesterol in Adults: Executive summary of the third report of the National Cholesterol Education Program (NCEP) Expert Panel on Detection, Evaluation, and Treatment of High Blood Cholesterol in Adults. *Journal of the American Medical Association, 285,* 2486-2497. Available at www.guideline.gov/algorithm/2778/FTNGC-2778.html.

American Heart Association. (2002). Cholesterol-lowering drugs-AHA recommendation. Retrieved January 25, 2004, from www.americanheart.org.

Bojar, R.M. (1992). *Adult cardiac surgery.* Cambridge, MA: Blackwell Scientific Publications.

Bonser, R.S., Quinn, D.W., & Harrington, D.K. (2003). The prediction of thoracic aneurysm expansion. In D. Liotta, M., et al. (Eds.). *Diseases of the aorta* (2nd ed., pp. 156-181.). Buenos Aires, Argentina: University of MoRón.

Charanjit, R.S., et al. (2003). Indications for coronary artery bypass surgery and percutaneous coronary intervention in chronic stable angina. *Circulation, 108*(20), 2439-2451.

Chobanian, A.V., et al. (2003). Seventh report of the Joint National Committee on prevention, detection, evaluation and treatment of high blood pressure. *Hypertension, 42,* 1206-1252.

David, J.L., & Limet, R. (1999). Antiplatelet activity of clopidogrel in coronary artery bypass grafting surgery patients. *Thrombosis Haemostasis, 82*(5), 1417-1421.

Del Rio, M., Liotta, D., & Gallo, A. (2003a). The clinical aspects of degenerative diseases and aneurysm of the aorta. In D. Liotta, et al. (Eds.). *Diseases of the aorta* (2nd ed., pp. 203-218.). Buenos Aires, Argentina: University of MoRón.

Del Rio, M., & Liotta, D. (2003b). Etiology, pathogenesis, and clinical aspects of aortic dissection. In D. Liotta, et al. (Eds.). *Diseases of the aorta* (2nd ed., pp. 219-242). Buenos Aires, Argentina: University of MoRón

Foley, K.A., et al. (2003). Development and validation of the hyperlipidemia. *Journal of General Internal Medicine, 18*(12), 984-990.

Khan, N.E., et al. (2004). A randomized comparison of off-pump and on-pump multivessel coronary-artery bypass surgery. *The New England Journal of Medicine, 350*(1), 21-28.

Pericarditis. (2001-2003, April 7, 2003). Retrieved January 25, 2004, from www.OHSU.edu.com.

Reid, N. (2003). Heart center online for cardiologists and their patients: Pericarditis. Retrieved January 9, 2004 from www.heartcenteronline.com.

Selnes, O.A., et al. (2003). Cognitive changes with coronary artery disease: A prospective study of coronary artery bypass graft patients and nonsurgical controls. *Annals of Thoracic Surgery, 75,* 1377-1386.

U.S. Department of Health and Human Services; National Institutes of Health; National Heart, Lung, and Blood Institute. (2003). The Seventh Report of the Joint National Committee on Prevention, Detection, Evaluation, and Treatment of High Blood Pressure. NIH Pub. No. 03-5233. Bethesda, MD: Author.

Van Dijk, D., et al. (2002). Cognitive outcome after off-pump and on-pump coronary artery bypass graft surgery. *JAMA, 287*(11), 1405-1412.

Chapter 8

Gastrointestinal Disorders

Kathyrn L. Burg and Karen Campbell Betten

1. **What is the gastrointestinal (GI) differential diagnosis for acute epigastric pain?**
   - Perforated duodenal ulcer
   - Acute pancreatitis
   - Biliary colic (or right upper quadrant [RUQ])
   - Acute gastritis

2. **What is the GI differential diagnosis for acute lower quadrant pain?**
   - Acute appendicitis (initially presents as poorly localized periumbilical pain then moves to the right lower quadrant [RLQ])
   - Acute mechanical obstruction of the colon, which can occur throughout both lower quadrants
   - Acute diverticulitis (left lower quadrant [LLQ])

3. **What are the most common GI causes of acute upper quadrant pain?**
   - Acute cholecystitis (RUQ/epigastric)
   - Acute mechanical obstruction (small bowel): can be periumbilical or throughout both upper quadrants

4. **What symptoms and presentation would be associated with a perforated duodenal ulcer?**
   - *Presenting symptoms*: sudden onset of pain and nausea
   - *Description of pain*: sharp, intense pain, often preceded by gnawing, aching, burning pain
   - *Location of pain*: epigastric region, often radiating to the back and spreading throughout the abdomen if peritonitis develops
   - *Associated symptoms*: tachycardia, fever, hypotension, tachypnea

5. **What first steps are taken in the evaluation of a patient with suspected perforated duodenal ulcer?**
   - Physical examination
   - Abdominal computed tomography (CT) scan
   - Laboratory studies: complete blood count and serum chemistries

6. **Describe the clinical presentation of a patient with suspected pancreatitis.**
   - *History*: often significant for weight loss, anorexia, and nausea.
   - *Presenting symptoms*: steady pain in the epigastric region, often radiating to the back. Lying supine often exacerbates pain; sitting up with trunk flexed can alleviate the severity of the pain. Patients often appear to be in distress.
   - *Associated symptoms*: tachycardia, hypotension.
   - *Laboratory studies*: elevated serum amylase and white blood cell (WBC) count.

7. **What is biliary colic?**

   Biliary colic is an acute obstruction of the cystic or common bile duct, usually caused by cholelithiasis.

8. **How does biliary colic present?**
   - *History*: associated with anorexia, nausea, vomiting, and weight loss. Onset of pain often occurs 15 to 60 minutes after a meal.
   - *Presenting symptoms*: jaundice, steady, achy epigastric, RUQ abdominal pain. Pain often radiates to the right shoulder and scapula. Pain has a rapid onset, lasts a few hours, gradually subsides, and is often recurrent.
   - *Associated symptoms*: nausea, dyspepsia, and flatulence. Bilious vomiting is common and subsides as the pain improves.
   - Temperature is usually normal and WBC count is not elevated.

9. **What abnormal diagnostic findings are present with biliary colic?**
   - Abdominal ultrasound usually reveals cholelithiasis.
   - Liver function tests show elevated alkaline phosphatase and direct bilirubin.

10. **What is acute cholecystitis?**

    Acute cholecystitis is an acute inflammation of the gallbladder usually caused by the blockage of the cystic duct by a gallstone.

11. **In the acute care setting, what patients are more likely to develop cholelithiasis?**

    Cholelithiasis can occur in patients on total parental nutrition (TPN) because the gallbladder becomes enlarged due to a lack of the hormonal stimulation that accompanies oral feeding. Similarly patients who are critically ill and unable to take oral feedings can develop gallbladder stasis, which can lead to accumulation of toxic agents in the gallbladder lumen, causing inflammation and acute cholecystitis.

12. **What symptoms of acute cholecystitis are different from those of biliary colic?**
    - Acute onset of pain in the RUQ, often radiating to the right scapula or shoulder (of longer duration than with biliary colic)
    - Often associated with fever and elevated WBC count

13. **What is the workup for acute cholecystitis?**
    - Abdominal ultrasound reveals gallstones, gallbladder wall thickening, and a positive Murphy's sign.
    - HIDA/Nuclear medicine scan reveals nonvisualization of the gallbladder.
    - WBC count is elevated.

14. **The patient is vomiting bile. How can one tell if the patient has a small bowel obstruction?**
    - *History*: previous abdominal surgery, which may create adhesions and increases potential for hernias.
    - *Presenting symptoms*: sudden onset of cramping, colicky periumbilical or upper abdominal pain. Pain is worse when obstruction occurs in the jejunum. Severity of pain decreases as bowel motility diminishes. Patients are often restless.
    - *Vomiting* of bile and mucus is indicative of a high obstruction. Vomiting fecal material is indicative of a low obstruction.
    - *Obstipation* gradually develops.
    - *Physical examination*: high-pitched, hyperactive bowel sounds. Tenderness to palpation is not impressive, unless leakage of small bowel contents has occurred.

15. **What diagnostic studies should be initially performed in a patient with suspected small bowel obstruction?**
    - Abdominal radiograph study
    - CT scan of the abdomen with contrast

16. **What is the initial treatment for a small bowel obstruction?**

    The initial treatment for a small bowel obstruction is to place a nasogastric tube to decompress the bowel.

17. **What complications are particularly associated with bariatric surgery?**
    - *Anastomotic leak* occurs at the connection between the new small stomach pouch and the small intestine (roux-en-Y limb). This causes bile to leak into the peritoneum and may result in infection.
    - *Strictures* can occur at the anastomosis between the pouch and intestine as well. A stricture is a tightening of the opening, resulting in nausea, vomiting, and possible dehydration.
    - Patients who are obese and who are immobile following surgery are at increased risk for *deep vein thrombosis* and *pulmonary embolus*.

18. **What is the initial treatment for complications associated with bariatric surgery?**
    - When the *anastomotic leak* is small, patients are given nothing by mouth (NPO). TPN and intravenous (IV) acid suppression is administered. If the leak is large, reoperation may be required.

- For a *stricture*, diagnosis and treatment occur during endoscopy. If a stricture exists, it can be dilated during the procedure.
- To prevent *deep vein thrombosis*, all patients should receive subcutaneous heparin and compression stocking following surgery. If any symptoms of leg pain, edema or cramping occur, suspicion of embolus should be immediate. This is also true of sudden onset of tachycardia, tachypnea, and desaturation. In the postoperative bariatric surgery patient, pulmonary embolus should be ruled out immediately. Treatment of suspected pulmonary embolus includes IV heparin, oral warfarin (Coumadin) therapy and, often, placement of an inferior vena cava (IVC) filter.

19. What is an upper GI bleed?

An upper GI bleed refers to bleeding proximal to the ligament of Treitz that leads to hematemesis, hematochezia, or melena.

20. What is a lower GI bleed?

Lower GI bleeds occur distal to the ligament of Treitz (junction between the duodenum and the jejunum). The color of blood is associated with the length of time the blood is in the GI tract. Bleeding distal to the ligament of Treitz is characterized by dark to bright red blood from the rectum. The dark color is a result of the oxidation of heme by bacterial and digestive enzymes.

21. What information helps hone in on the correct diagnosis?

- Note any recent episodes of GI bleeding.
- Note any known conditions that predispose the patient to GI bleeding.
  - Recent surgery
  - Liver disease
  - History of gastric or duodenal ulcers
  - Thrombocytopenia
  - Uremia
  - von Willebrand's disease
- Note any medications that predispose to bleeding.
  - Heparin
  - Warfarin
  - Aspirin
  - Nonsteroidal anti-inflammatory drugs
  - Steroids

22. After taking the history and completing a thorough physical examination, what are the first steps in managing GI bleeding?

- Begin assessment with the ABCs (airway, breathing, circulation) including hemodynamic stability and degree of blood loss.
- Establish venous access with two large-bore catheters.

- Send blood for analysis of complete blood count, prothrombin time, partial thromboplastin time, platelet count, and type and cross-match.
- Consider applying a Foley catheter to monitor volume status.
- Begin fluid resuscitation as necessary.
- A nasogastric (NG) tube can be placed to rule out an upper GI source.
- Anoscopy, digital rectal examination, or rigid proctosigmoidoscopy can be done to rule out anorectal disease.
- An esophagogastroduodenoscopy (EGD) can be done to rule out an upper GI source.
- Obtain a surgical consult when indicated.

23. **What are the most frequent causes of upper GI bleeding?**
- Acute gastritis
- Duodenal ulcer
- Gastric ulcer
- Mallory Weiss tear
- Esophageal or gastric varices

24. **How can the source of bleeding be identified in an upper GI bleed?**

An esophagogastroduodenoscopy (EGD) is considered the most useful diagnostic procedure to evaluate the source of bleeding. The timing of endoscopy is often a matter of clinical judgment based on available resources and the character and severity of the bleeding. Angiography with intra-arterial infusion of vasopressin or embolization can be effective if the bleeding site can be visualized. If stabilization is unsuccessful, operative intervention may be indicated.

25. **What is the differential diagnosis for lower GI bleed?**
- Bleeding vascular ectasias
- Diverticular bleeding
- Colon cancer
- Colonic polyps
- Ischemic colitis
- Infectious colitis
- Inflammatory bowel disease
- Anorectal disorder (hemorrhoids, rectal fissures)
- Meckel's diverticulum

26. **What options are available to localize the source of lower GI bleeding?**
- *Colonoscopy* can establish a definite or probable diagnosis in more than 80% of individuals with lower GI bleeding.
- *Angiography* detects bleeding at a rate of 0.5 mL/min.
- *Sulfur colloid scan* detects bleeding rates as low as 0.05 to 0.10 mL/min.
- *Tagged red blood cell scan* detects bleeding rates as low as 0.05 to 0.10 mL/min.

27. **In what percentage of patients does lower GI hemorrhage spontaneously resolve?**

Lower GI bleeding resolves in 75% of patients with vascular ectasias and 90% of patients with diverticular bleeding.

28. **What is diverticulosis?**

Diverticulosis is an outpouching of the mucosa and submucosa through the muscular layers of the bowel wall. It can occur anywhere in the colon. In the United States, 95% of all cases of diverticulosis occur in the left colon, primarily the sigmoid colon. However, diverticulosis occurs more commonly in the right colon in Japanese and Chinese patients.

29. **What is diverticulitis?**

Diverticulitis refers to the inflammation and infection of the diverticula. Only 10% to 15% of patients with diverticulosis develop diverticulitis. Diverticulitis is most common in the sixth or seventh decade of life. Patients younger than 50 years of age tend to have more complications.

30. **Can diverticular disease cause bleeding?**

Yes. Diverticulosis is one of the most common causes of lower GI bleeding. However, bleeding from diverticulitis is uncommon.

31. **What are the most common clues to diagnosing diverticulitis?**

Evaluation of Diverticulitis

Evaluation	Findings
History	Fever and chills, alteration of bowel habits, documented diverticulosis
Pain	Severe achy, crampy pain; left lower quadrant (LLQ) greater than right lower quadrant (RLQ)
Examination	LLQ tenderness
Studies	Elevated white blood cell count. Computed tomography scan may show colonic inflammation, abscess, or mass if perforation has occurred.

32. **What complications are associated with diverticulitis?**

Perforation of diverticulum can result in any of the following:
- Intra-abdominal abscess
- Peritonitis
- Fistula to the bladder, vagina, or skin from the diseased colon
- Bowel obstruction

33. **What is the best test for diagnosing acute diverticulitis or perforation?**

Abdominal CT scan with rectal contrast is advocated by most hospitals for diagnosing both diverticulitis and perforation. Typical findings include diverticulitis with inflammatory thickening of the bowel wall.

34. **What is the most common treatment for acute diverticulitis?**
   - Fluid resuscitation
   - Pain management
   - Antibiotics
   - NPO or clear fluid

If localized abscess is found, CT-guided percutaneous drainage is indicated. Emergency surgical management is reserved for perforation with impending sepsis; however, if the patient is hospitalized, surgical consultation is advisable.

35. **Describe the differences in clinical presentation and management of acute large bowel obstruction and acute small bowel obstruction (SBO).**

Small Bowel Obstruction versus Large Bowel Obstruction

	Small Bowel Obstruction	Large Bowel Obstruction
Pain	Sudden diffuse, intermittent cramping immediately after meals or 1 hr postprandially.	Intermittent crampy lower quadrant pain not associated with meals.
Emesis or stool	***Vomiting*** Clear fluid indicates gastric contents. Green fluid is from the duodenum and jejunum. Bilious or golden fluid indicates bile duct entry into bowel. Feculent fluid from near cecum where bacteria have decomposed bowel fluid. ***Stool*** Watery diarrhea from proximal SBO. No stool once distal tract is emptied from distal SBO.	May have fullness and bloating. ***Vomiting*** Rare until late in the process. ***Stool*** Obstipation; alternating diarrhea and constipation may indicate a partial obstruction.
Physical examination	Mild diffuse abdominal tenderness. High-pitched tinkling bowel sounds. Old abdominal incision. Low-grade fever. Dehydration. Low urine output.	Abdominal distention. High-pitched bowel sounds with rushes. May progress to silence with localized tenderness (indicating peritonitis). Rectal mass may be palpable. Stool may be positive for blood in cases of tumor.

Continued

Small Bowel Obstruction versus Large Bowel Obstruction—cont'd

	Small Bowel Obstruction	Large Bowel Obstruction
Workup	Blood tests: complete blood count and serum electrolytes. Abdominal series may show dilated loops of small bowel or air-fluid levels. Typically the colon distal to the obstruction is empty of gas and stool. Upright chest radiograph if perforation is suspected.	Blood tests: complete blood count and serum electrolytes. Arterial blood gas if patient has respiratory compromise due to distention or diaphragmatic compression. Abdominal series typically shows dilated loops of bowel or air-fluid levels. The proximal small bowel is normal if the ileocecal valve is competent. A cecum measuring greater that 10 to 12 cm is an indication of impending perforation. Upright chest radiograph if perforation is suspected. Proctoscopy or colonoscopy may reveal a mass. Contrast enema may be necessary for full evaluation.
Most common causes of obstruction	Adhesions from prior abdominal surgery. Incarcerated or strangulated hernia. Neoplasm. Inflammatory bowel disease.	Mechanical • Carcinoma • Volvulus • Diverticular disease Less common mechanical • Hernias • Intussusception • Benign tumors • Fecal impaction Nonmechanical • Toxic megacolon • Paralytic ileus • Pseudo-obstruction
Treatment	Nothing by mouth (NPO). Nasogastric (NG) decompression. Fluid and electrolyte management. Intravenous antibiotic in the setting of fever, leukocytosis, or evidence of perforation. Emergent surgical management for evidence of perforation.	NPO. NG decompression. Fluid and electrolyte management. Intravenous antibiotic in the setting of fever, leukocytosis, or evidence of perforation. Emergent surgical management for evidence of perforation. Colonoscopy or sigmoidoscopy may be necessary for decompression (i.e., volvulus).

Key Points

- When differentiating types of epigastric pain, it is important to obtain an accurate history of presenting symptoms in order to implement the appropriate diagnostic workup.
- The three most common and serious complications associated with bariatric surgery are anastomotic leak, stricture, and deep vein thrombosis.
- When managing GI bleeding, it is imperative to understand how to differentiate between upper and lower GI sources of bleeding.

Internet Resources

American College of Gastroenterology:
www.acg.gi.org

GastroHep.com (access to some information requires $100 subscription):
www.gastrohep.com

Bibliography

Adams, G., & Bresnick, S. (1997). *On call surgery*. Philadelphia: W.B. Saunders.

Cho, K.C., et al. (1999). Sigmoid diverticulitis: Diagnostic role of CT—Comparison with barium enema studies. *Radiology, 176*, 111-115.

Howden, C. (2003, October). Emergency room and inpatient care: Options for immediate treatment. In *Optimizing the management of upper gastrointestinal bleeding: From emergency room to community.* (Section 3). Retrieved February 24, 2004, from www.medscape.com/viewarticle/463190_2.

Liscum, K. (1996). Lower gastrointestinal bleeding. In A. Harken & E. Moore (Eds.). *Abernathy's surgical secrets* (3rd ed., pp. 166-167). Philadelphia: Hanley & Belfus.

Nicoll, D., et al. (Eds.). (1997). *Pocket guide to diagnostic tests*. Stamford, CT: Appleton & Lange.

Norton, L.W. (2000). Diverticular disease of the colon. In A. Harken & E. Moore (Eds.). *Abernathy's surgical secrets* (3rd ed., pp. 157-158). Philadelphia: Hanley & Belfus.

Shelton, B. (1999). Intestinal obstruction. *AACN Clinical Issues, 10*, 478-491.

Terdiman, J. (2001). Colonoscopic management of lower gastrointestinal hemorrhage. *Current Gastroenterology Rep, 5*, 425-432.

Waring, J. (2002). Surgical and endoscopic treatment of GERD. *Gastroenterology Clinics of North America, 31*, 89.

Chapter 9

Neurological Disorders

Angela M. Votodian and Jean Dougherty Luciano

1. **What is a seizure?**

   A seizure is a temporary alteration in the electrical activity of the brain.

2. **Describe the classification of seizures.**

Seizure Classification		
Partial (Focal)	**Simple Partial**	**Complex Partial**
Consciousness is normal.	Symptoms may be motor, auditory, or sensory.	Confused purposeless behavior may be associated.
	No change in consciousness.	Impaired alertness and responsiveness sometimes preceded by an aura and followed by a postictal state.

3. **Describe a generalized seizure.**

   A generalized seizure is a sudden stiffness lasting a few seconds, followed by a rhythmic muscle contraction during the clonic phase that is followed by a postictal phase.

4. **What is the most common type of generalized seizure?**

   The most common type of generalized seizure is a grand mal seizure

5. **What are important questions to ask when evaluating a patient with seizures?**
   - Have you ever experienced head injury?
   - Have you ever had meningitis or encephalitis?

   If patient has a known seizure disorder:
   - When was your last seizure?
   - How often do they occur?
   - Are there other associated symptoms, auras, or incontinence?

- How long do the seizures last?
- Have you ever injured yourself or others during a seizure?

6. **What are common causes of seizures?**
   - Space-occupying lesions
   - Encephalitis
   - Subarachnoid hemorrhage (SAH)

7. **What diagnostic studies should be ordered when evaluating a patient with seizures?**
   - Computed tomography (CT), magnetic resonance imaging (MRI), or both
   - Electroencephalography (EEG)
   - Laboratory tests: complete blood count (CBC), serum electrolytes, liver panel, and serum glucose

8. **What are treatment options for seizures?**
   - Antiepileptic drugs
   - Surgery, an option for patients who fail pharmacologic therapy

9. **What are common causes of a hemorrhagic stroke?**
   - Nontraumatic injury
   - Cerebral aneurysm
   - Hypertension
   - Vascular malformations
   - Brain tumors
   - Bleeding diathesis

10. **Which aneurysm is associated with sustained hypertension?**

    Charcot-Bouchard aneurysm is associated with sustained hypertension.

11. **What are the types of cerebral aneurysms?**
    - Saccular
    - Intracranial arterial dissection
    - Infective
    - Neoplastic
    - Traumatic

12. **What are the types of vascular malformations?**
    - Arteriovenous malformation
    - Telangiectasis
    - Cavernous angioma
    - Venous angioma

13. **What are the treatment options for vascular malformations?**
    - Surgical resection
    - Embolization of vessels
    - Stereotactic administration of high-density radiation

14. **What clinical conditions are associated with intracerebral hemorrhage (ICH)?**
    - Thrombocytopenia
    - Leukemia
    - Hemophilia A or B
    - Sickle cell disease

15. **Which pharmacological agents or drugs may cause an ICH?**
    - Thrombolytic agents
    - Anticoagulants
    - Aspirin
    - Cocaine
    - Amphetamines

16. **What common symptoms are associated with ICH?**
    - Worst headache of life
    - Syncope
    - Nausea and vomiting

17. **What common signs are associated with ICH?**

    The common signs associated with ICH are third nerve palsy with diminished light reflex and pupillary dilation.

18. **What historical questions are important in the evaluation of a patient with suspected ICH?**
    - Do you have a headache?
    - Do you have visual changes?
    - Do you have motor or speech difficulties?
    - Do you have other comorbid medical conditions?
    - Do you have a history of thrombotic conditions?
    - Are you taking medications?
    - Are you on anticoagulant or aspirin therapy?
    - Do you have a family history of aneurysms?

19. **What diagnostic studies should be obtained in the evaluation of ICH?**
    - Noncontrast brain CT
    - Lumbar puncture
    - CBC

- Chemistry panel
- Hepatic function panel
- Prothrombin time (PT), activated partial thromboplastin time

20. What is the emergency management for patients with intracranial bleeding?

Therapeutic intervention is based on decreasing the volume of the hematoma and preventing cell death. Therefore acute interventions should focus on reversing and controlling the source of bleeding and managing increased intracranial pressure. The goal is to reduce clot volume after the hematoma has expanded:

- Most important, address the ABCs (airway, breathing, and circulation).
  - Intubation protects the airway and permits hyperventilation (to decrease ICP)
- Use medical management to reverse causes of active bleeding (fresh frozen plasma [FFP], vitamin K, platelets).
- Blood pressure control is of key importance (a systolic blood pressure of less than 160 is acceptable at most institutions).
  - Labetalol and nicardipine are commonly used.
- Patients should be in a neurointensive care unit.
- Frequent neurological assessments are made using the Glasgow coma score.
- ICP monitoring with the use of a fiberoptic intraparenchymal monitor or ventriculostomy can be used to reduce ICP.
- Neuroradiological procedures include clipping and coiling.
- Surgical intervention depends on the following:
  - Age of the patient
  - Size and the location of the bleed

21. List general treatments of a subarachnoid hemorrhage.

- Bed rest, dark quiet environment
- Opiates for headaches
- Thermoregulation: keep normothermic or hypothermic
- Antiemetics
- Anticonvulsants
- Treatment of vasospasm with calcium channel blockers (amlodipine)
- Treatment of increased ICP and hydrocephalus with mannitol

22. What are the types of strokes?

- Ischemic stroke: may be thrombotic or embolic (approximately 80%)
- Hemorrhagic stroke (approximately 20%)

23. What are common manifestations of stroke?

Acute development of a focal neurological deficit. The deficits depend upon the area of ischemia or hemorrhage. They may include motor or sensory loss, aphasia, dysarthria, facial weakness, body neglect, vertigo, ataxia, headache, and visual impairment such as field cut, blindness, or diplopia.

24. **What are the key questions in history taking?**
    - What are the date and time of the onset of the symptoms?
    - Do you have any risk factors for stroke such as hypertension, cardiac disease or dysrhythmia, diabetes, hypercholesteremia, or a hypercoagulable state?
    - Do you have a personal or family history of stroke or transient ischemic attack?

25. **What are the key elements of the acute phase clinical assessment?**
    - Vital signs, medical history, history of current event, physical examination, and neurological examination
    - Noncontrast head CT scan
    - Blood glucose, CBC with differential, platelet count, PT, partial thromboplastin time, serum chemistries
    - 12-lead electrocardiogram

26. **Describe the management of the patient with an acute stroke?**
    - For acute stroke patients with onset of symptoms of less than 3 hours (and meeting all other inclusion/exclusion criteria), intravenous recombinant tissue plasminogen activator (rt-PA) should be considered. If rt-PA is given, strict adherence to protocol for post rt-PA patient management is essential. Note especially the blood pressure management and the restrictions for the use of antithrombotic and antiplatelet agents.
    - For positioning for ischemic stroke, keep the head of bed flat. For hemorrhagic stroke patients, keep the head of bed at approximately 30 degrees.
    - All patients should be kept normovolemic with isotonic fluids; avoid dextrose.
    - Maintain normothermia or hypothermia; use acetaminophen as indicated.
    - Maintain mean arterial pressure of 70 to 150 mm Hg.

27. **What diagnostic studies may be ordered in the evaluation of a patient with an acute stroke?**
    Customize your evaluation according to the patient's age, history, risk factors, location of the stroke, and findings from previous studies to streamline the evaluation. The evaluation may include any part of the following:
    - MRI, MR angiography, CT angiography (CTA), conventional angiogram
    - Transthoracic or transesophageal echocardiogram
    - Carotid and vertebral duplex ultrasounds
    - Blood toxicology screen, sedimentation rate, hematologic studies

28. **What are the common primary brain tumors?**
    - Astrocytoma
    - Oligodendroglioma
    - Glioblastoma multiforme (most common)

29. **What is the common clinical presentation of a patient with a primary brain tumor?**

  * Headache (usually worse after arising)
  * Tinnitus, unilateral hearing loss, vertigo (acoustic schwannoma)
  * Seizures
  * Motor deficit

30. **How are brain tumors diagnosed?**

  * Brain biopsy is the definitive diagnosis and allows for histological staging.
  * Head CT scan can identify brain tumors.

31. **What cerebrospinal fluid (CSF) findings may be present in patients with brain tumors?**

  * Elevated pressure
  * Elevated protein

32. **What are the treatments for patients with brain tumors?**

  * Steroids (Decadron) to control cerebral edema
  * Anticonvulsants to control seizures
  * Surgical resection (curative or palliative)
  * Radiation and gamma knife
  * Chemotherapeutic agents

33. **What pathogens are responsible for meningitis?**

  * Bacterial
  * Fungal
  * Viral

34. **What are the most common bacterial pathogens responsible for meningitis?**

  * *Streptococcus pneumoniae*
  * *Neisseria meningitidis*
  * *Haemophilus influenzae*
  * *Escherichia coli*
  * *Listeria monocytogenes*

35. **What are predisposing factors for the development of meningitis?**

  * Systemic infection
  * Head trauma
  * Neurological procedures
  * Cancer
  * Alcoholism
  * Immunodeficiency

36. **What manifestations are commonly associated with meningitis?**
    - Nuchal rigidity
    - Headache
    - Fever
    - Vomiting
    - Confusion
    - Seizures

37. **What two clinical signs are associated with meningitis?**
    - The Kernig sign
    - The Brudzinski sign

38. **What is the Kernig sign?**

    Kernig sign, a clinical hallmark of meningitis, is elicited by having the person lie supine, flex the thigh so it is at a right angle to the trunk, and completely extend the leg at the knee joint. If the leg cannot be completely extended due to pain, this is Kernig sign.

39. **What is the Brudzinski sign?**

    The Brudzinski sign is positive when flexion of the neck causes flexion of the legs at the knees, hips, and ankles.

40. **Describe the different CSF findings in patients with bacterial, viral, and fungal meningitis.**

Cerebrospinal Fluid Findings in Different Types of Meningitis			
	Bacterial	**Viral**	**Fungal**
White blood cell count	Increased neutrophils	Mildly elevated	Moderately elevated
Glucose	Decreased	Normal	Normal
Protein	Increased	Mildly elevated	Mildly elevated

41. **What is the most common cause of fungal meningitis in the immunodeficient patient?**

    The most common cause of fungal meningitis in the immunodeficient patient is *Cryptococcus*.

42. **What is the usual treatment for cryptococcus meningitis?**

    Amphotericin B is the usual treatment for cryptococcus meningitis.

43. What is the most common cause of encephalitis?

Herpes simplex virus type 1 (HSV-1) and arbovirus are the most common causes of encephalitis.

44. How is encephalitis characterized?

- It is characterized by inferior frontal and temporal lobes.
- Manifestations are similar to meningitis but with a more gradual onset.
- In herpes encephalitis, frontal and temporal symptoms may result in personality changes and memory loss.

45. What tests are helpful in the diagnosis of HSV encephalitis?

- Lumbar puncture: CSF findings are similar to those for viral meningitis, that is, high opening pressure, elevated WBC count (lymphs), presence of RBCs, increased protein, normal glucose
- EEG: periodic lateralizing epileptiform discharges
- MRI: the preferred imaging study; pathologic changes in medial temporal and inferior frontal areas
- Polymerase chain reaction (PCR): analysis of CSF
- Brain biopsy: role of brain biopsy is decreasing with advent of PCR technology

46. What is the management for viral encephalitis?

- Treatment for HSV encephalitis is intravenous acyclovir.
- Control of headache and fever are of key importance.
- Osmotic diuretics may be used in the event of cerebral edema.
- Anticonvulsants can be given for seizure prophylaxis.

Key Points

- Hypertension is a leading cause of stroke and intracerebral hemorrhage.
- Nuchal rigidity is commonly associated with meningitis.
- A normal EEG does not exclude epilepsy.

Internet Resources

E-Medicine Textbooks: Neurology:
www.emedicine.com/neuro/contents.htm

Journal Watch Neurology:
neurology.jwatch.org

Biology Online: Neurology Tutorial:
www.biology-online.org/tutorials/8_neurology.htm

Bibliography

Devinsky, O., Feldman, E., & Weinreb, H. (2000). *Neurologic pearls.* Philadelphia: F.A. Davis.

Logan, P. (1999). *Principles of practice for the acute care nurse practitioner.* Stamford, CT: Appleton & Lange.

Miller, J., & Fountain, N. (1997). *Neurology recall.* Philadelphia: Williams & Wilkins.

Pouratian, N., Kassell, N., & Dumont, A. (2003). Update on management of intracerebral hemorrhage. *Neurosurgical Focus* 15(4). Available at www. aans.org/education/journal/neurosurgical/oct03/15-4-2.pdf.

Tierney, L., McPhee, S., & Papadakis, M. (2000). *Current medical diagnosis and treatment* (39th ed.). New York: McGraw-Hill.

Chapter 10

Renal and Genitourinary Disorders

Eunice N. Jeon

1. What is the etiology of hematuria?

Common causes include urinary tract infection (UTI), stones, trauma, malignancies of the bladder or kidney, benign prostatic hyperplasia, and postoperative hematuria. Less common causes include adverse effects of medication, exercise-induced hematuria, radiation or chemical cystitis, sickle cell anemia, vascular disease, coagulopathy, and glomerulonephritis.

2. What is the workup for a patient who presents with hematuria?

Once the diagnosis of hematuria is established by history and physical as well as a urine analysis, UTI must first be ruled out. If the patient's hematuria is due to a UTI, most patients do not need a further workup. The UTI can be treated and no catheter is needed as long as the patient can empty his or her bladder. Medication use and coexisting medical problems should also be evaluated as potential causes. Treatment should begin with hydration and consultation with a urologist for further evaluation of the cause of hematuria and to rule out any malignancies. If renal calculi is suspected, the patient should be instructed on straining urine and hydration.

3. What is the significance of hematuria in relation to its timing during urination?

The timing of when bleeding occurs during urination can indicate where the probable site of bleeding is. When bleeding occurs at the beginning of the urinary stream, anterior urethral bleeding may be indicated. Terminal hematuria that occurs only at the end of the stream can indicate bleeding from the posterior urethra, bladder neck, or trigone. If the hematuria occurs throughout the entire stream, it indicates that the bleeding is originating from the bladder or above.

4. How does a patient with nephrolithiasis present?

- Paroxysmal pain lasting 20 to 60 minutes
- Nausea and vomiting
- Microscopic or gross hematuria
- Dysuria

- Urinary frequency and urgency
- Pain may radiate to other areas such as groin or back

5. **What tests can be used in the evaluation of nephrolithiasis?**

- Urinalysis. A low pH (<5.5) may be present with uric acid stones and a high pH (>7.2) may be present with struvite stones. Hematuria as well as white blood cells may be detected.
- Urine culture can detect a concurrent UTI.
- KUB (plain film of the kidneys, ureters, and bladder). Most stones are radiopaque and can be detected by the KUB, except stones composed of pure uric acid. Size, number, and location can also be detected.
- IVP (intravenous pyelogram). This is the diagnostic procedure of choice and can detect radiolucent stones. If the patient is allergic to dye, he or she may be premedicated with steroids and Benadryl.
- US (ultrasonography). Although the sensitivity of this test is less than that of a radiograph, this is the procedure of choice for patients who are pregnant or who have a known allergy to contrast medium.
- CT (computed tomography) scan. This test also has a high sensitivity and specificity for stones.

6. **Under what conditions is hospitalization of a patient with nephrolithiasis required?**

- Pain that cannot be controlled with oral medications
- Patient has only has one kidney and presents with anuria or presents with a urethral stone that is obstructive, larger than 6 mm, and may need to be treated with a therapeutic procedure
- Syncopal episodes

7. **How does a patient with acute pyelonephritis present?**

- Fever
- Chills
- Flank pain
- Costovertebral angle tenderness
- About 75% of patients admit to a recent history of a lower UTI
- Urinalysis is positive for white blood cells, bacteria, and white cell casts
- Lower urinary tract symptoms such as dysuria, frequency, and urgency

8. **What is the treatment for acute pyelonephritis?**

Eighty percent of pyelonephritis is caused by *Escherichia coli*. Therefore, in an uncomplicated case, oral fluoroquinolones can be administered for 7 days or trimethoprim-sulfamethoxazole can be given for 14 days. If the patient presents with sepsis, vomiting, dehydration, or a complicated case of pyelonephritis caused by conditions such as urinary obstruction, urinary tract abnormalities, or an immunocompromising condition, a hospital stay is warranted with the administration of parenteral antibiotic therapy. After the initial treatment with parenteral antibiotics, the clinically stable patient (as defined by a normal blood pressure and ability to keep fluids down) may be converted to oral antibiotic therapy as an outpatient.

9. **What is the etiology of urinary retention?**

Urinary retention is most commonly caused by benign prostatic hypertrophy, but it can also be caused by urethral stricture, contracture of the bladder neck, postoperative pain, medication side effects, or neurological diseases.

10. **How should a patient with urinary retention be managed?**

The placement of an average-sized Foley catheter (18 Fr) should be attempted. If this fails, in a patient with benign prostatic hypertrophy (BPH), the insertion of a larger, coudé-tipped catheter may be attempted after inserting lubricating jelly into the urethra. In a patient with urethral strictures or contractures of the bladder neck, a smaller catheter (e.g., 12 or 14 Fr) can be used. If these attempts fail, a urologist should be consulted.

11. **What are the corresponding laboratory findings and expected compensation in acid-base disorders?**

Corresponding Laboratory Findings and Expected Compensation in Acid-Base Disorders

Disorder	pH	Primary Defect	Compensatory Response
Respiratory acidosis	↓pH	↑P_{CO_2}	↑HCO_3^- by 0.1 mEq/L for each ↑ 1 mm Hg of P_{CO_2}
Respiratory alkalosis	↑pH	↓P_{CO_2}	↓HCO_3^- by 0.25 mEq/L for each ↓ 1 mm Hg of P_{CO_2}
Metabolic acidosis	↓pH	↓HCO_3^-	↓P_{CO_2} by 1.25 mm Hg for each ↓ 1 mEq/L of HCO_3^-
Metabolic alkalosis	↑pH	↑HCO_3^-	↑P_{CO_2} by 0.2-0.9 mm Hg for each ↑ 1 mEq/L of O_3^-

12. **How should the acid-base status of a patient be determined?**

- Determine the main acid-base disorder by evaluating the arterial laboratory values.
- Evaluate the possibility of a mixed acid-base disorder by determining whether or not the degree of compensation for the main disorder is appropriate.
- Evaluate the patient's manifestations and determine whether or not they correlate with the acid-base analysis.

13. **What are the subclassifications of acute renal failure?**

- *Prerenal:* a reversible syndrome that is caused by transient, poor renal perfusion due to volume depletion, decrease in cardiac output, or redistribution of extracellular fluid. In this condition, the kidney's structure and function remain normal.
- *Postrenal:* a syndrome that is caused by an obstruction in the urinary tract. As the obstructed urine accumulates, the back pressure that is built causes renal tubular dysfunction that produces urine that has an increased urine sodium level and fractional excretion of sodium (FENa).
- *Intrinsic:* a syndrome that is caused by four conditions:
  - *Acute tubular necrosis:* a condition that occurs as a result of an ischemic or toxic injury to the kidney
  - *Acute glomerulonephritis:* a condition that occurs when the glomeruli become inflamed, resulting in a decrease in the glomerular blood flow as well as a decrease in the glomerular filtration rate
  - *Allergic interstitial nephritis:* a condition that is caused by a reaction to a variety of drugs
  - *Large vessel occlusion:* a rare condition that is caused by the occlusion of one of the major renal arteries or veins in a patient with only one functioning kidney

14. **What does a urinalysis show in acute renal failure?**

Urinalysis Results in Acute Renal Failure

	Prerenal	AGN	ATN	Obstruction
Urine osmolarity (mOsm/kg H_2O)	>350	>350	<350	<350
Urine sodium level (mEq/L)	<30	<30	>30	>30
Qualitative urine protein	Negative to trace	3 to 4+	Trace to 2+	Negative to trace
Urine microscopic sediment	Normal	Red cells/ casts	Normal	Normal
Fractional excretion of sodium	<1%	<1%	>1%	>1%

From P.M. Hanno, S.B. Malkowicz, & A.J. Wein (Eds.). (2001). *Clinical manual of urology* (3rd ed., p. 477). New York: McGraw-Hill.
AGN, Acute glomerulonephritis; *ATN,* acute tubular necrosis.

15. **What is the definition of chronic renal failure (CRF)?**

CRF is diagnosed when the acute injury that initially caused renal failure does not resolve and there is a persistent abnormality in the glomerular filtration rate (GFR), resulting in the destruction of functioning nephrons.

16. **How should a patient who is in renal failure who needs a study requiring intravenous (IV) contrast be managed?**

    IV saline hydration, reduction of contrast used, and use of acetylcysteine (600 mg by mouth, twice a day before and on the day of the contrast study) can help reduce the nephrotoxicity of IV contrast dye.

17. **What commonly used drugs can cause acute interstitial nephritis leading to acute renal failure?**
    - Nonsteroidal anti-inflammatory drugs (NSAIDs)
    - Penicillins, cephalosporins
    - Rifampin
    - Sulfonamides
    - Cimetidine
    - Allopurinol
    - Ciprofloxacin
    - 5-Aminosalicylates

18. **How is glomerulonephritis diagnosed?**

    A urinalysis with the findings of proteinuria, hematuria, and red blood cell casts are the classic signs of glomerulonephritis.

19. **How should a patient with glomerulonephritis be evaluated?**

    To identify the cause of glomerulonephritis, a comprehensive serologic evaluation should be performed to test for the presence of systemic vasculitis, collagen vascular disease, or any type of infectious process. A renal biopsy should also be performed.

 Key Points

- Any patient who presents with hematuria that is not attributed to a UTI must be referred to a urologist to rule out any potential malignancies.
- Many commonly prescribed classes of drugs, including antimicrobials and NSAIDs, can cause acute renal failure.
- A complicated case of pyelonephritis may warrant hospitalization and parenteral administration of intravenous antibiotics.

Internet Resources

Digital Urology Journal:
www.duj.com/unohome

Kidney & Urology Foundation of America, Inc.:
www.kidneyurology.org

Medical Information Organization: Urology Section:
urology.medical-information.org

Bibliography

Bloom, R.D., & Grossman, R.A. (2001). Renal physiology: Acute and chronic renal failure. In P.M. Hanno, S.B. Malkowicz, & A.J. Wein (Eds.). *Clinical manual of urology* (3rd ed., Chapter 16). New York: McGraw-Hill.

Blumenfeld, J.D., & Vaughan, E.D. (2002). Renal physiology and pathophysiology. In P.C. Walsh, et al. (Eds.). *Campbell's urology* (8th ed., pp. 214-220). Philadelphia: W.B. Saunders.

Fukagawa, M., Kurokawa, K., & Papadakis, M.A. (2001). Fluid & electrolyte disorders. In L.M. Tierney, S.J. McPhee, & M.A. Papadakis (Eds.). *Current medical diagnosis & treatment* (40th ed., pp. 885-888). New York: McGraw-Hill.

Forget, S., et al. (2003). Calculous renal failure and pregnancy. *Progres en Urologie 13*(4), 673-674.

Goldfarb, D.A., Nally, J.V., & Schreiber, M.J. (2002). Etiology, pathogenesis, and management of renal failure. In P.C. Walsh, et al. (Eds.). *Campbell's urology* (8th ed., p. 275). Philadelphia: W.B. Saunders.

Greenstein, A., et al. (2003). Is intravenous urography a prerequisite for renal shockwave lithotripsy? *Journal of Endourology, 17*(10), 835-839.

Hochreiter, W., Knoll, T., & Hess, B. (2003). Pathophysiology, diagnosis and conservative therapy of non-calcium kidney calculi. *Therapeutische Umschau Revue Therapeutique 60*(2), 89-97.

Ianenko, E.K., et al. (2003). Urinary tract occlusion: A principal cause of some complications of urolithiasis. *Urologiia, Feb.* 28(1), 17-21.

Kawashima, A., & LeRoy, A.J. (2003). Radiologic evaluation of patients with renal infections. *Infectious Disease Clinics of North America, 17*(2), 433-456.

Kim, J. (2004). Ultrasonographic features of focal xanthogranulomatous pyelonephritis. *Journal of Ultrasound Medicine, 23*(3), 409-416.

Kohn, I.J., & Weiss, J.P. (2001). Pyelonephritis. In P.M. Hanno, S.B. Malkowicz, & A.J. Wein (Eds.). *Clinical manual of urology* (3rd ed., Chapter 8). New York: McGraw-Hill.

Kunin, C.M. (1997). *Urinary tract infections: Detection, prevention, and management* (5th ed., pp. 190-198). Baltimore: Williams & Wilkins.

Menon, M., & Resnick, M.I. (2002). Urinary lithiasis: Etiology, diagnosis, and medical management. In P.C. Walsh, et al. (Eds.). *Campbell's urology* (8th ed., pp. 3267-3277). Philadelphia: W.B. Saunders.

Pahira, J.J., & Razack, A.A. (2001). Nephrolithiasis. In P.M. Hanno, S.B. Malkowicz, & A.J. Wein. *Clinical manual of urology* (3rd ed., Chapter 9). New York: McGraw-Hill.

Prince, J.S., & Senac, M.O. Jr. (2003). Ceftriaxone-associated nephrolithiasis and biliary pseudolithiasis in a child. *Pediatric Radiology, 33*(9), 648-651.

Rabii, R., et al. (2003). Symptomatic bladder calculi: Diagnostic and therapeutic aspects. *Annales d'Urologie (Paris). 37*(3), 93-95.

Schaeffer, A.J. (2002). Infections of the urinary tract. In P.C. Walsh, et al. (Eds.). *Campbell's urology* (8th ed., pp. 551-553). Philadelphia: W.B. Saunders.

Shinghal, R., & Payne, C.K. (2001). Emergency room urology. In P.M. Hanno, S.B. Malkowicz, & A.J. Wein (Eds.). *Clinical manual of urology* (3rd ed., Chapter 10). New York: McGraw-Hill.

Tepel, M., et al. (2000). Prevention of radiographic-contrast-agent-induced reductions in renal function by acetylcysteine. *New England Journal of Medicine, 343*(3), 180-184.

Yilmaz, E., et al. (2003). C-Reactive protein in early detection of bacteriemia and bacteriuria after extracorporeal shock wave lithotripsy. European Urology, *43*(3), 270-274.

Chapter 11

Musculoskeletal and Vascular Disorders

Annemarie Murphy

MUSCULOSKELETAL PROBLEMS

1. What is gout?

Gout is an inflammatory disease, which classically presents as an acute mono-arthritis. This inflammation typically affects the peripheral joints and is a reaction to monosodium urate (MSU) crystals.

2. What is the classic presentation of gout?

Typically, men older than age 30 are affected most. The disease does not usually affect women until their postmenopausal years. Gout can occur acutely or chronically.

ACUTE PHASE
The acute phase frequently occurs at night or early morning and the pain peaks with 24 to 36 hours. The pain is characteristically severe and is accompanied by joint inflammation and fever. The most common location of an acute flare-up is the first metatarsophalangeal joint of the great toe. If left untreated, symptoms may resolve in a few days to weeks.

CHRONIC PHASE
During the chronic phase of gout, asymptomatic periods become less frequent and more joints are involved. Joints of the feet, ankles, wrists, hands, and elbows are affected. As the disease progresses, symptoms such as morning stiffness, joint tenderness, a low-grade fever, and swelling from the accumulation of tophi in joints, bursae, and subcutaneous tissues are exacerbated.

3. How is gout diagnosed?

The most favorable way to diagnose gout is by the presence of MSU crystals in the synovial fluid or a tophus. Tophi are accumulations of MSU in soft tissue.

Although serum uric acid levels are typically elevated in patients with gout, it is often improperly used in making a diagnosis of gout. A uric acid level greater than 7.0 mg/dL supports a diagnosis of gout; however, chronic use of certain medications such as aspirin and diuretics can also elevate uric acid levels. Older adults may also have hyperuricemia and never develop gout.

4. What diagnostic studies help in the accurate diagnosis of gout?

- Aspirate joint fluid and send a culture and smear to identify MSU and to rule out an infection.
- Obtain a uric acid level.
- A 24-hour urinalysis measures uric acid levels; normal values are 600 to 900 mg.
- Sedimentation rates and white blood cell counts are elevated during an acute attack.

5. What are the treatment options for an episode of acute gout?

Nonsteroidal anti-inflammatory drugs (NSAIDs) are the best choice during an acute flareup of gout. A high dosage of these medications should be used with a gradual reduction of the dose when symptoms subside. Effective NSAIDs for an acute flareup of gout are Naprosyn or Indocin.

For individuals who cannot tolerate NSAIDs, colchicine should be considered. However, colchicine must be avoided in individuals with hepatic or renal insufficiency.

6. What are treatment options for chronic gout?

To prevent or relieve chronic gout, uric acid levels must remain stable. To avoid fluctuation in uric acid levels, allopurinol is often the urate lowering agent of choice.

7. Are there standard findings in the clinical diagnosis of rheumatoid arthritis (RA)?

Yes. The American Rheumatology Association has classified certain criteria necessary for the diagnosis of RA. Of the following criteria, four must be present for the diagnosis to be made. These criteria are as follows:
- Morning stiffness, for 6 months, which takes a minimum of an hour to dissipate.
- Arthritis of at least three or more joints for 6 months
- Arthritis of hand joints for 6 months
- Symmetric arthritis for 6 months
- Rheumatoid nodules
- Rheumatoid factor in serum
- Radiological changes

8. What laboratory tests should be ordered?

A complete blood count (CBC) with differential, erythrocyte sedimentation rate, urinalysis, and rheumatoid factor titer should be obtained for baseline information in individuals in whom RA is suspected.

9. **What are the goals of treatment and management for RA?**

There is no cure for RA, but the treatment goals are to relieve pain, to maintain joint function, and to prevent disease progression. Interventions such as the administration of disease-modifying agents, anti-inflammatory medications, and physical therapy exercises can help achieve these treatment goals. The management of RA is challenging because of the self-limiting, disabling, and chronic components of the disease.

10. **What is osteoarthritis (OA)?**

OA is a musculoskeletal disease characterized by the degeneration of articular cartilage of joints and dense bone formation at the base of cartilage lesion.

11. **Are there risk factors associated with OA?**

Yes. Factors that may contribute to the development of OA include obesity, age, joint trauma, occupational overuse, muscle weakness, estrogen use, and genetics. Congenital musculoskeletal, metabolic, or endocrine disorders could also contribute to the development and progression of OA.

12. **What are the specific characteristics of OA?**

The onset of OA is often slow with a gradual development of joint pain, effusions, deformity, and crepitus. Morning stiffness occurs, but unlike RA the stiffness typically dissipates within 30 minutes.

13. **How is OA treated?**

Similar to RA, there is no cure for OA. However, the treatment goals for OA are to control pain and to keep the current level of functioning in the patient's routine activities of daily living. The classic treatment for OA usually combines one or more oral medications with exercise. For pain control, acetaminophen is typically used as first-line therapy. The daily dosage of acetaminophen should not exceed 4 g. For individuals who do not get relief from acetaminophen, the next option is a low dose of NSAIDs. If an individual cannot tolerate NSAIDs because of gastrointestinal side effects, cyclooxygenase-2-specific inhibitors (COX-2) medications can be used. However, COX-2 inhibitors have been associated with an increased risk of cardiovascular complications. Rofecoxib (Vioxx) was withdrawn from the market in the latter part of 2004 because of concern for these risks.

14. **What are the risk factors for osteoporosis?**

- Female gender
- Low body weight (<58 kg)
- Physical inactivity
- Menopause
- Bilateral oophorectomy
- Heredity

- Low calcium/vitamin D intake
- Smoking

15. Can the intake of calcium delay the occurrence of osteoporosis?

Yes. The daily recommended amount of calcium (see the following table) would increase mineral bone density, therefore possibly decreasing the risk of developing or delaying the onset of osteoporosis.

Daily Recommended Amounts of Calcium

AGE (yr)	DAILY CALCIUM REQUIREMENTS
9-18	1300 mg
19-50	1000 mg
50+	1200 mg (for men and women who are taking hormone replacement) 1500 mg (for women who are not taking hormone replacement)

16. What studies should be ordered to help diagnose osteoporosis?

A dual-energy x-ray absorptiometry (DEXA) scan is the most reliable study for diagnosing osteoporosis. After the diagnosis of osteoporosis is made, a DEXA scan should be completed every 2 years. The best way to predict fractures is to measure the density of the proximal femur. The best way to assess the effectiveness of treatments is to measure the density of the lumbar spine. Determining an individual's bone mineral density (BMD) is another way to diagnose osteoporosis. The BMD can be measured using the hip, spine, or forearm. The World Health Organization supports a diagnosis of osteoporosis if the BMD is 2.5 or more standard deviations below the mean of a healthy individual of the same gender and age group.

17. What is compartment syndrome?

Compartment syndrome is an abnormal increase in tissue pressure within a closed anatomical space. With this dangerous increase in tissue pressure, perfusion of the muscles is compromised and, if left untreated, can lead to ischemia and functional impairment.

18. What is considered a high intracompartmental pressure?

When intracompartmental pressures increase to 30 mm Hg or greater, tissue perfusion is impaired and an intervention is necessary. If this increase in pressure is not recognized, the patient is at risk for tissue necrosis and possible limb loss. Normal capillary perfusion pressure averages 25 mm Hg.

19. **What causes compartment syndrome?**

    Compartment syndrome occurs because the pressure is too high. This harmful increase in pressure is attributed to an increase in fluid content or a decrease in compartment size. Increased amounts of fluid can be caused by burn injuries, intensive muscle use, hemorrhage, and decreased serum osmolarity. A decrease in compartment size can arise after a burn injury and a cast placement.

20. **What symptoms are associated with compartment syndrome?**
    - Extreme pain after an injury to an extremity (at rest or with any movement)
    - Burning and tightness in the area of the injury
    - The traditional 5 "*P's*": pain, paraesthesia, pallor, poikilothermia, pulselessness

21. **What is the differential diagnosis for compartment syndrome?**
    - Cellulitis
    - Gas gangrene
    - Necrotizing fasciitis
    - Peripheral vascular injuries
    - Rhabdomyolysis
    - Deep vein thrombosis
    - Phlebitis

VASCULAR PROBLEMS

22. **What is deep vein thrombosis?**

    Deep vein thrombosis (DVT) is a formation of a blood clot in the deep venous system. The etiology of DVT is unknown, even though Virchow's triad of blood stasis, injury to the vessel wall, and hypercoagulability are key components to the development of DVT.

23. **How does a patient with DVT present?**

    Generally, a patient with DVT presents with swelling, localized pain, tenderness, redness, and warmth.

24. **What are the risk factors for developing DVT?**
    - Sedentary lifestyle
    - Prolonged bedrest
    - Immobility (especially after a long airplane trip)
    - Obesity
    - Recent surgery (particularly orthopedic, gynecologic, or heart surgery)
    - Fractures or trauma to the lower extremities
    - Malignant tumors
    - Pregnancy

25. What diagnostic studies should be ordered to help confirm the diagnosis of DVT?

A venous Doppler, magnetic resonance venography (MRV), or contrast venography can confirm the diagnosis of DVT. If there is a suspicion of pulmonary compromise, a $\dot{V}/\dot{Q}$ scan should be ordered to help rule out a pulmonary embolism.

26. What are treatment options for DVT?

Anticoagulants should be started immediately and the patient should elevate the affected limb for comfort. The anticoagulant helps prevent further clots from forming and worsening the current condition. A Greenfield filter may be placed in the inferior vena cava (IVC) if a patient cannot be anticoagulated or if the patient has persistent thrombotic events despite adequate anticoagulation. This intervention helps prevent a pulmonary embolism.

27. How does superficial phlebitis differ from DVT?

Superficial phlebitis affects the veins closer to the skin surface. Superficial phlebitis is generally not as severe as DVT, and with proper care it will dissipate quickly and without intervention.

28. What is the typical presentation of superficial phlebitis?

Superficial phlebitis has a gradual onset and the area is usually tender and warm. There is often a thin, red area of inflammation that frequently can be palpated. When palpable, the vein feels like cords.

29. What is the treatment for superficial phlebitis?

Typically there is no medical or surgical treatment for superficial phlebitis. The patient should be instructed to keep the area clean. Warm soaks may aid in alleviating any pain or discomfort.

30. What are common complications of a superficial phlebitis and DVT?

- Pulmonary embolism
- Repeat thrombosis (superficial or deep)
- Venous stasis ulcers

31. What is a venous stasis ulcer?

A venous stasis ulcer is the most common lesion on the lower extremity. This troublesome type of ulcer often occurs in the presence of chronic venous insufficiency. A venous stasis ulcer can follow DVT that was complicated by the disruption of blood flow between the deep and superficial venous system. A minor traumatic event to a chronically swollen leg can also cause a venous stasis ulcer.

32. **Does a venous stasis ulcer hurt?**

Yes. A patient with a venous stasis ulcer often complains of increased discomfort or pain when the affected leg is dependent. The pain is often times alleviated with elevation.

33. **What is the clinical presentation of a venous stasis ulcer?**

The ulcer itself is typically shallow with exudate covering the base of the wound. The edges are irregular and the surrounding skin thick and hyperpigmented. Arterial blood flow is usually unaffected in the presence of a venous stasis ulcer; therefore although the lower extremity is edematous, pulses are often palpable.

34. **Describe the treatment plan for a venous stasis ulcer.**

Elevation to control the swelling is crucial in this type of wound healing. The wound cannot contract if the leg is constantly swollen. To facilitate this necessary compression, an Unna boot (a medicated bandage) or a surgical support stocking may need to be prescribed for the patient.

Debridement may be required if there is an increase in exudate that will impede wound contraction. This can be accomplished mechanically or enzymatically. Topical agents, such as calcium alginate, hydrocolloid, or hydrogel can be applied to the wound to aid in healing. Antibiotic creams should be avoided because these creams can exacerbate stasis dermatitis and prevent wound healing.

If a venous stasis ulcer is not showing signs of improvement within 4 to 6 weeks, consider a wound biopsy and refer the patient to a wound care specialist.

35. **What is intermittent claudication?**

Intermittent claudication is an early manifestation arterial insufficiency. Claudication symptoms occur in individuals with compromised blood flow to certain muscle groups. The primary symptom of pain often occurs with exercise and is relieved with rest. The location of the pain or discomfort is dependent upon the location of the vascular disease. The symptoms can be unilateral or bilateral.

If a patient suffers from aortoiliac disease, he or she will most likely complain of claudication symptoms in the buttock, hip, and thigh region. A complaint of thigh claudication often indicates occlusions of the femoral arteries. Calf claudication is the most common claudication complaint. If the symptoms occur in the upper portion of the calf, the stenosis is usually in the superficial femoral artery. If the symptoms occur in the lower portion of the calf, the stenosis is most likely in the popliteal artery.

36. **What are the risk factors for developing claudication symptoms?**

- Diabetes mellitus
- Hypertension

- Tobacco use
- Hyperlipidemia

37. What diagnostic tests that can be performed to aid in determining the diagnosis of arterial insufficiency?

Pulse volume recordings (PVRs) with an ankle-brachial index (ABI) can help determine the degree of disease. An MRA scan can also be a helpful study to provide a roadmap of the blockages in the legs. An arteriogram is an invasive study that can be performed if symptoms are debilitating to the patient.

38. How is arterial insufficiency treated?

The main objective to treating arterial insufficiency and claudication symptoms is to control the patient's risk factors. Smoking cessation, antihypertensives, and lipid management may help with symptoms. An arteriogram with possible angioplasty of the stenotic lesions may also aid in symptom relief.

39. What is cellulitis?

Cellulitis is an acute infection of the skin and subcutaneous tissues. This infection can occur in any part of the body, although it is mostly seen on an extremity.

40. What is the clinical presentation of cellulitis?

- Warm, red, swollen skin
- Tender skin
- Fever
- Malaise
- Chills
- Lymphadenopathy

41. Is cellulitis ever an emergency?

Yes. Cellulitis can develop into an emergency situation. Findings that signify an emergency situation include the following:
- Presence of cutaneous necrosis
- Fever, or other signs of septicemia
- Weak arterial pulses
- Extensive cellulitis
- Immunosuppressed or diabetic patient
- Necrotizing cellulitis

42. What is the treatment for cellulitis?

If the infection is uncomplicated, oral antibiotics for 10 to 14 days is an appropriate treatment plan. In an emergent situation, hospitalization is required with intravenous (IV) antibiotic therapy. The antibiotics may have to be changed secondary to culture results and lack of clinical response.

For all cases, whether emergent or not, nonpharmacological measures should be used. For example, elevation, immobilization, and the application of warm compresses to the affected area may aid in symptomatic relief.

43. What is a necrotizing infection?

Necrotizing infections can occur in the skin and fascia in the form of necrotizing cellulitis and fasciitis. Necrotizing fasciitis is an infection of the subcutaneous tissue that slowly destroys the fascia and fat. However, this type of infection may not affect the skin.

44. How does necrotizing fasciitis present?

The progression of the disease is typically rapid and therefore early recognition is crucial. The first sign of the disease is typically unexplained pain that quickly intensifies with no sign of any skin irritation. Erythema usually develops within 2 days of the pain along with fever, malaise, myalgias, anorexia, and diarrhea. The erythema can be diffuse or local and darken to a deep purple with blisters and bullae. The presence of bullae typically indicates deep soft tissue involvement.

45. What tests can be ordered to help make the diagnosis of narcotizing fasciitis?

- Hematology panel: leukocytosis
- Cardiac panel: elevated serum creatinine kinase and creatinine concentrations
- Cultures: blood and wound
- Radiological studies: presence of gas in the tissue and/or soft tissue swelling

46. How is necrotizing fasciitis treated?

The most beneficial treatment of necrotizing fasciitis is surgical exploration and debridement of the necrotizing tissue. In addition to this intervention, IV antibiotics and hemodynamic support may also be required.

 Key Points

- The treatment goal for RA is to prevent disease progression and disability.
- Deep vein thrombosis management is aimed at preventing the development of pulmonary embolism.
- The development of a compartment syndrome is considered an emergency.

Internet Resources

DVT.net:
dvt.net

National Institute of Arthritis and Musculoskeletal and Skin Diseases (NIAMS):
www.niams.nih.gov

Health Resources on the Web: Vascular Disorders:
www.cytos.org/vascular-disorders.html

Bibliography

Bickley, L.S., & Hoekelman, R.A. (1999). *Bates' guide to physical examination and history taking* (7th ed.). Philadelphia: Lippincott Williams & Wilkins.

Gorrol, A.H., & Mulley, A.G. (2000). Primary care medicine (4th ed.). Philadelphia: Lippincott Williams & Wilkins.

Uphold, C.R, & Graham, M.V. (1999). *Clinical guidelines in adult health* (2nd ed.). Gainesville, FL: Barmarrae Books.

Chapter 12

Hematological and Oncological Disorders

Colleen M. Harker

1. What are the three physiologic causes of anemia?

- Excessive blood loss
- Inadequate production of red blood cells (RBCs)
- Excessive destruction of RBCs

2. What are the most common types of anemia, their causes, and treatments?

Common Types of Anemias

	Diagnosis	Causes	Treatment
Iron-deficiency anemia	Absent bone marrow iron stores or serum ferritin ≤12 mcg/L	Decreased production of red blood cells (RBCs) Increased destruction of RBCs Extrinsic hemolysis	Oral iron (FeSO$_4$ 325 mg three times daily). Parenteral iron (used for intolerance of oral iron, gastrointestinal disease, and continued blood loss. The dose is calculated by supplying 1 mg of iron for each milliliter of volume of RBC count below normal).
Anemia of chronic disease	Low serum iron, normal or increased serum ferritin, low total iron binding capacity (TIBC)	Chronic infection or inflammation Cancer Liver disease	In most cases, no treatment is necessary. RBC transfusion for those who are symptomatic. Purified recombinant erythropoietin has been shown to be effective at a dose of 10,000 units injected subcutaneously three times weekly.

Continued

Common Types of Anemias—cont'd

	Diagnosis	Causes	Treatment
Vitamin B_{12} deficiency	Macrocytic anemia Hypersegmented neutrophils on peripheral blood smear Serum vitamin B_{12} level <100 pg/mL	Dietary deficiency Decreased production of intrinsic factor Pancreatic insufficiency Decreased ileal absorption of vitamin B_{12}	Intramuscular injections of 100 mcg of vitamin B_{12} given daily for the first week, weekly for the first month, and then monthly for life.
Folic acid deficiency	Macrocytic anemia Hypersegmented neutrophils on peripheral blood smear Normal serum vitamin B_{12} levels Reduced folate levels in red blood cells or serum	Dietary deficiency Decreased absorption (tropical sprue; drugs such as phenytoin, Bactrim) Increased requirement (chronic hemolytic anemia, pregnancy, exfoliative skin disease) Loss: dialysis Inhibition of reduction to active form (methotrexate)	Folic acid 1 mg/day orally.
Sickle cell anemia	Irreversibly sickled cells on peripheral blood smear Positive family history and lifelong history of hemolytic anemia Recurrent painful episodes Hemoglobin S (the major hemoglobin seen on electrophoresis)	An autosomal recessive disorder with abnormal hemoglobin levels related to chronic hemolytic anemia and having many clinical consequences	Folic acid supplementation. Transfusions for aplastic or hemolytic crises. Pneumococcal vaccinations reduce the incidence of infections. With exacerbations, patient should be kept well hydrated, and oxygen should be given. Acute vaso-occlusive crises can be treated with exchange transfusions.
Aplastic anemia	Pancytopenia No abnormal cells seen Hypocellular bone marrow	Congenital (rare) Idiopathic (autoimmune) Systemic lupus erythematosus Chemotherapy; radiotherapy Toxins: benzene, toluene, insecticides Some drugs Post-hepatitis Pregnancy	Largely symptomatic, based on avoiding exposure to cold. Alkylating agents such as chlorambucil for severe involvement. High-dose IV immuno-globulin (2 g/kg) and interferon may be of some benefit.

3. **What signs are seen in a patient with compensated anemia?**

Although most patients are asymptomatic, they may have an increased heart rate, increase cardiac output, or increased stroke volume.

4. **What are the manifestations of uncompensated anemia?**

- Lethargy
- Exertional dyspnea
- Dizziness
- Headache
- Systolic murmur (in some patients)
- "Thumping palpitations" related to high output
- High-pitched tinnitus
- Postural faintness or syncope

5. **What aspects of a patient's clinical history are important to obtain when evaluating suspected anemia?**

- Abnormal blood loss
- Change in bowel habits
- Melena or hematochezia
- Aspirin or anticoagulant use
- Family history of anemia
- History of malignancy
- Chronic inflammatory process
- Pica
- Dysphagia
- Lead exposure
- Menstrual blood loss
- Gastric resection or colonic resection (in past 2 to 4 months)
- Change in nails or nailbeds

6. **What is the primary problem that leads to manifestations of leukemia?**

The uncontrolled proliferation of one (or more) types of hematopoietic cells (lymphocytes, granulocytes, monocytes, or erythrocytes) or a precursor or these cells. This uncontrolled proliferation occurs at any point in the cycle of cell maturation.

7. **What are the two classes of leukemia and how are they differentiated?**

Acute leukemias, including acute lymphoblast leukemia (ALL) and acute myelogenous leukemia (AML), involve undifferentiated or immature cells and are rapid in onset and progression. If untreated, acute leukemias typically are associated with a life expectancy of only days to months.

Chronic leukemias, including chronic myelogenous leukemia (CML) and chronic lymphoblastic leukemia (CLL), have a gradual onset and prolonged progression and clinical course. Life expectancy is typically greater than 10 years, and although symptoms and disease state are easily controlled by conventional chemotherapy, this treatment, in most cases, does not prolong life expectancy.

8. **How is spinal cord compression (SCC) defined and which malignancies are most likely to cause this complication?**

   SCC is the displacement, compressive indentation, or enclosure of the spinal cord's thecal sac by metastatic or locally aggressive cancer, causing edema, inflammation, and mechanical compression of the spinal cord itself and leading to direct neural injury, vascular damage, and decreased oxygenation. Patients at highest risk for development of SCC by metastatic tumor are those with lung cancer, breast cancer, prostate cancer, cancer of unknown origin, and renal cancer, although any invasive cancer with hematogenous spread can cause SCC.

9. **What clinical presentation would alert one to the possibility of SCC?**

   Although the presenting manifestations depend on the level of the spine affected, the cardinal initial symptom in most patients is pain that precedes other symptoms by approximately 2 to 4 months. Pain may be local, caused by vertebral destruction by an enlarging tumor mass, or radicular, caused by compression of surrounding nerve roots. Other symptoms that be discovered during physical examination are as follows:
   - Soreness or tenderness over the vertebral body (point tenderness)
   - Muscle weakness or paresis
   - Gait problems
   - Bilateral leg weakness, especially noticeable with stair climbing
   - Paresthesias in one or both legs
   - Change in bowel or bladder habits
   - Decreased sensory function
   - Weak rectal sphincter tone (late sign)
   - Urinary retention related to neurogenic bladder (late sign)

10. **How is SCC compression diagnosed?**

    Diagnosis is based on physical examination and diagnostic testing as follows:
    - *Plain spine radiograph* demonstrates associated vertebral blastic or lytic lesions.
    - *Magnetic resonance imaging (MRI) of the spine* gives the health care practitioner the most definitive view of spinal lesions and shows cord compression caused by extradural masses as well as paravertebral masses, intramedullary disease, and bone metastasis.

11. **What is the treatment of SCC?**

    - Treatment is palliative in most cases, with the goals being relief of pain and maintenance and restoration of neurological function.

- Corticosteroids, such as dexamethasone, reduce the associated edema and cord compression, thereby decreasing pain. (Adult dose ranges from 4 to 100 mg, given every 6 hours, based on the weight of the patient.)
- Radiation therapy is the standard of care, resolving pain by reducing tumor mass and relieving the SCC. Indications of response are decreased pain and return to baseline function or improvement of function.
- In some patients with spinal instability or rapid progression, surgery may be indicated to alleviate pressure.
- Patients should always have spinal immobilization, pain control, close skin assessment, and monitoring of bowel and bladder habits while undergoing treatment for SCC.

12. What is superior vena cava (SVC) syndrome?

SVC syndrome, most often associated with lung cancer, breast cancer, and lymphomas, is due to the obstruction by thrombosis or direct tumor invasion of the SVC or by collapse from tumor compression extrinsically. Other causes are mediastinal or radiation fibrosis and thrombosis, most often associated with a central access line.

13. What is the clinical presentation in patients with SVC syndrome?

The presentation of SVC is related to poor venous return, increased intravenous pressure, and collateral vessel engorgement. Manifestations include the following:
- Facial swelling
- Truncal and extremity swelling
- Dyspnea
  - Chest pain
  - Cough
- Dysphagia
- Dizziness
  - Syncope
  - Visual disturbances
- Thoracic vein distention
  - Neck vein distention
  - Tachypnea
- Plethora of face
- Cyanosis

14. How is SVC diagnosed?

This is a clinical diagnosis, based on clinical manifestations. Chest computed tomography (CT) may be useful in localizing the mass and in suggesting other complications that may arise, but it is not diagnostic. Chest radiograph is abnormal in approximately 80% of patients and illustrates superior mediastinal masses, pleural effusions, or right upper lobe masses in most patients with abnormalities.

15. How is SVC syndrome treated?

Patients with evidence of tracheal compression or stridor should be approached as true emergencies and treated immediately. Nonspecific methods should be used to decrease venous pressure, including bedrest with reverse Trendelenburg position, diuretics, decreased sodium intake, and supplemental oxygen. Emergent radiation may be lifesaving in patients with tracheal compression.

16. What are the major presenting symptoms for patient with malignant pericardial disease?

- Pulsus paradoxus
- Venous hypotension
- Narrow pulse pressure
- Tachycardia
- Shock, only if cardiac tamponade is severe, presenting with facial swelling, dyspnea, and nonspecific chest discomfort

17. How would a patient with cardiac tamponade caused by malignant pericardial disease be treated?

- Intravenous volume expansion
- Supplemental oxygen
- Pericardiocentesis to relieve pressure and obtain cells for definitive diagnosis
- Indwelling intrapericardial catheters in conjunction with intrapericardial administration of sclerosing agents (e.g., doxycycline or bleomycin) to prevent further symptomatic recurrence
- Surgical approaches, such as subxiphoid pericardial window, limited thoracotomy with pericardial window, or thoracotomy with pericardiectomy, in patients with a reasonable expected survival

18. What are the components of neutropenic precautions?

- Strict handwashing is the most important precaution for all persons who touch the patient.
- It is not necessary for health care providers to wear masks, but those who have signs or symptoms of a respiratory disease should not come in contact with the patient. The practice of requiring patients to wear masks when in the hallway varies between institutions.
- There should be positive airflow in the patient's room as compared to the hallway. The intent is to avoid exposure to airborne pathogens.
- The patient's room should be cleaned so as to not cause dust to be shed.
- Sources of gram-negative organisms should be avoided (e.g., fruits and vegetables, live flowers, and raw food).

19. When should neutropenic precautions be implemented?

Neutropenic precautions should be implemented when the white blood cell (WBC) count becomes dangerously low, because neutropenia is the single most important factor in determining whether a cancer patient will become infected.

The absolute neutrophil count (ANC) is calculated by multiplying the percentage of granulocytes (neutrophils or segments + bands) by the total WBC count. The risk of infection rises as the WBC count falls, with the greatest risk at neutrophil counts less than 500/mm³. Most serious infections occur once neutrophil counts fall below 100/mm³.

20. When is fever in neutropenic patients significant?

In the presence of neutropenia, fever is always significant and should be treated as a medical emergency. A prompt and effective therapy must begin within hours because the patient is in mortal danger. In neutropenic patients, fever is almost always a sign of bacteremia. Clinical evidence of infection and systemic inflammatory response are usually equated with sepsis, especially in patients with proven neutropenia.

Most authorities agree that significant fever in the neutropenic patient is a single oral temperature greater than or equal to 38.5° C (101° F) in the absence of a clear cause or the presence of a temperature greater than 38° C (100.4° F) for 1 hour or more.

21. What is the treatment of a patient with neutropenic fever?

Empirical antibiotic therapy should begin as soon as appropriate cultures, namely blood, urine, stool, sputum, and wound sites, are obtained. It is also appropriate and necessary to obtain a chest radiograph to evaluate for pneumonia. If any sign of sinus disease arises, a CT scan of the sinuses should be obtained, because plain radiographs are not effective in evaluating these infections.

In addition to these diagnostic tests, the following should be evaluated:
- Vital signs
- Mentation
- Urine output
- Platelet count
- Glucose

22. What physical assessment is important in patients with neutropenia and fever?

Physical Assessment of Neutropenia and Fever

System	Assessment Concentration
Skin	Assess for change in current or previous IV sites. Assess for new rashes that could be attributed to drug reaction or bloodborne spread of bacteria or fungi. Assess perianal pain or inflammation, considering hemorrhoids, fissure, or phlegmon (inflammation of soft tissue due to infection).

Continued

Physical Assessment of Neutropenia and Fever—cont'd

System	Assessment Concentration
Head and neck	Headache, sinus or jaw pain: consider sinusitis. Nasal ulcers or mucosal necrosis: consider fungal involvement. Cotton wool spots in front of retina: consider candida. Oral mucosal white patches that rub off and bleed: consider candida. Odynophagia (painful swallowing) with oral ulcers: consider herpes, thrush, or candida esophagitis.
Lungs	Findings on examination may be minimal as neutropenia may precede radiograph abnormalities.
Abdomen	Tenderness and rebound especially involving the right lower quadrant: consider appendicitis.

---

23. What is the syndrome of heparin-induced thrombocytopenia (HIT)?

HIT is an immune-mediated platelet activation, causing thrombocytopenia and endothelial release of thrombin in approximately 1% of all patients who receive unfractionated heparin, leading to intravascular thrombosis. The syndrome results from antibodies that activate platelets in response to heparin initiation, forming antigenic complexes that become targets for the antibodies formed. Formation of these complexes bind to circulating platelets and to heparin-like glycosaminoglycans on the surface of endothelial cells, causing platelet activation, platelet aggregation, and procoagulant platelet-derived microparticle formation and resulting ultimately in endothelial cell injury. This reaction causes a hypercoagulable state in which either arterial or venous thrombi develop in 30% to 80% of patients.

24. Describe the two separate types of HIT.

Heparin-Induced Thrombocytopenia

Type I (also called heparin-associated thrombocytopenia)	Type II
Nonimmune reaction	Immune-mediated response
Direct platelet activation, aggregation, and mild to moderate thrombocytopenia (usually >100,000 cells/μL).	Life- or limb-threatening thrombosis, severe thrombocytopenia (usually 30,000-55,000 cells/μL).
Occurs within hours of treatment initiation.	Occurs several days after therapy initiation.
Heparin therapy may continue.	Heparin therapy should be discontinued immediately.

Heparin-Induced Thrombocytopenia—cont'd

Type I (also called heparin-associated thrombocytopenia)	Type II
Treatment: observation.	Treatment: alternative anticoagulation and thrombin inhibitors.
Negative platelet aggregation test.	Positive platelet aggregation test in about 50% of cases.
Negative serotonin release assay.	Positive serotonin release assay in approximately 80% of cases.

25. What are the therapeutic options for anticoagulation in a patient with HIT?

- All sources of heparin should be immediately discontinued, including low-molecular-weight heparin, which has a 90% cross-reactivity to HIT antibodies.
- Other causes of thrombocytopenia should be ruled out before initiating therapy.
- Platelet transfusion should be reserved only for patients with risk of severe hemorrhage (platelet count < 20,000 cells/μL).
- Direct thrombin inhibitors, lepirudin, argatroban, and bivalirudin are available.
- Lepirudin and argatroban have a Food and Drug Administration approved indication for HIT. These have been shown to reduce the risk of death, amputation, and new thromboembolic complication when used in management of HIT. They are effective anticoagulants, inactivate both soluble and clot-bound thrombin, and do not cross-react with the HIT antibody. Both are administered by continuous intravenous (IV) therapy only.
- Bivalirudin is a potential treatment option, but should be reserved as the last option because limited data are available regarding its use.
- Caution should be taken when initiating warfarin therapy because activated partial thromboplastin time (aPTT) and international normalized ratio (INR) may increase rapidly and must be monitored closely.

🔑 Key Points

- Clinical manifestations of uncompensated anemia may appear long after a patient is considered clinically anemic by blood cell count values. When a patient begins to experience symptoms such as lethargy, dizziness, headaches, and shortness of breath, treatment must be initiated quickly.

Continued

Key Points *continued*

* Neutropenic precautions should be initiated for any patient with ANC <500/mm³. These precautions consist of the following:
  * Practice strict handwashing.
  * Any visitor or employee who has symptoms of respiratory disease must wear a mask while visiting the patient.
  * Patients must wear masks when outside their own room (this practice varies among institutions).
  * The patient's room must have a positive airflow as compared to the hallway.
  * All live flowers, raw foods, and fruits and vegetables should be avoided.
* Patients with HIT have the following therapeutic options when deciding upon treatment:
  * *All* sources of heparin should be discontinued immediately (including low-molecular-weight heparin).
  * Other causes of thrombocytopenia should be ruled out.
  * Platelet transfusion should only be initiated if the patient has a platelet count less than 20,000 cells/µL.
  * Direct thrombin inhibitors (lepirudin, argatroban, and bivalirudin) are available for use in treatment.
  * Coumadin (warfarin) should be initiated carefully, because INR may rise rapidly.

Internet Resources

American Society of Hematology:
www.hematology.org

Bloodline: Online Resource for Hematology Education and News:
www.bloodline.net

Laboratory Hematology: Official Journal of the International Society for Laboratory Hematology:
www.laboratoryhematology.com

Bibliography

Andrews, N.C. (1999). Disorders of iron metabolism. *New England Journal of Medicine, 341,* 1986.

Bunn, F.H. (1997). Pathogenesis and treatment of sickle cell disease. *New England Journal of Medicine, 340,* 762.

Carlson, R.W. (2002). Oncologic emergencies. WebMD Scientific American Medicine. Posted 12/1/02 at www.medscape.com/viewarticle/479305.

Corwin, H.L. (2003). Anemia in the critically ill. *Medscape Critical Care.* Posted 2/20/03 at www.medscape.com/viewarticle/449463.

Donovan, P.C. (2001). Heparin-induced thrombocytopenia: Strategies for identification and treatment. *Clinician Reviews, 93,*11.

Hiddemann, W., et al. (1999). Management of acute myeloid leukemia in elderly patients. *Journal of Clinical Oncology, 17,* 3569.

Osowski, M. (2002). Spinal cord compression: An obstructive oncologic emergency. *Topics in Advance Practice Nursing.* Posted 10/14/02 at www.medscape.com/viewarticle/442735.

Tong, L.M., & Mendez, M.N. (2002). Therapeutic considerations in the management of patients with heparin induced thrombocytopenia. *Progress in Cardiovascular Nursing, 142,* 17.

Yahalom, J. (1997). Oncologic emergencies. In V.T. DeVita, S. Hellman, & S.A. Rosenberg (Eds.). *Cancer principles and practice of oncology* (5th ed., p. 2469). Philadelphia, Lippincott-Raven.

Chapter 13

Health Promotion

Rosanne Iacono

1. What is the United States Preventive Services Task Force?

The U.S. Preventive Services Task Force is an independent panel of experts in primary care and prevention that systematically reviews the evidence and develops recommendations for clinical preventive services. The identification of specific preventive services that are appropriate for inclusion in periodic health visits has been one of the principal objectives of the U.S. Preventive Services Task Force Project.

2. What are the two overarching goals *Healthy People 2010* is designed to achieve?

- Increase quality and years of healthy life
- Eliminate health disparities

The *Healthy People 2010* initiative began from a 1979 report entitled "Healthy People: The Surgeon General's Report on Health Promotion and Disease Prevention." The goals of that report were not all achieved but it had such an impact that *Healthy People 2000* was established. *Healthy People 2000: National Health Promotion and Disease Prevention Objectives*, released in 1990, identified health improvement goals and objectives to be reached by the year 2000. The *Healthy People 2010* initiative continues in this tradition as an instrument to improve health for the first decade of the 21st century.

3. Screening measures are considered what type of prevention?

Screening is considered a form of secondary prevention because one aspect is to identify diseases such as diabetes and high blood pressure.

4. When should glaucoma screening be started in adults?

Glaucoma screening should begin for patients at age 40 and continue every 5 years until age 60, then it should be done every 2 to 3 years. Most people have no symptoms and no early warning signs. If open-angle glaucoma is not diagnosed and treated, it can cause a gradual loss of vision. This type of glaucoma develops slowly and sometimes without noticeable loss of sight for many years. It usually responds well to medication, especially if caught early and treated.

5. **When should a 50-year-old patient with a 5-year history of diabetes be instructed to have eye examinations?**

Instruct the patient to have an eye examination every year. The American Diabetes Association recommends dilated eye examinations yearly for adults with diabetes. The three primary vision complications of diabetes are retinopathy, cataracts, and possibly glaucoma. The risk of developing diabetes-related eye disease increases the longer a person has diabetes.

6. **Describe measures adults should take to help prevent gum and tooth decay.**

Regular dental care provider visits, flossing daily, brushing teeth daily with fluoride-containing toothpaste is recommended based on evidence of risk reduction from these interventions. There has not been any strong clinical evidence that chewing gum between meals prevents gum and tooth decay.

7. **Identify primary prevention measures for type 2 diabetes.**

The American Diabetes Association recommends at least 2 to 3 hours a week of moderate physical activity, maintaining a healthy weight, and eating a healthy low-fat diet to prevent type 2 diabetes. There is no evidence that either a nonfat or vegetarian diet decreases the risk for type 2 diabetes over a healthy low-fat diet.

8. **At what point should the discussion of osteoporosis begin in a 32-year-old woman?**

Education for prevention of bone loss should begin immediately. For prevention, include recommendations for exercise and appropriate calcium and vitamin D intake. Women begin to lose bone density in their 30s. The damage from osteoporosis begins early in life. Women reach peak bone density in their 30s and must take in enough calcium to build bones that will remain strong later in life.

9. **What risk factors increase the likelihood for developing osteoporosis?**

The National Osteoporosis Foundation has identified the following risk factors that increase the likelihood of developing osteoporosis:
- Female gender
- Thin or small frame
- Advanced age
- Family history of osteoporosis
- Status postmenopause, including surgically induced menopause
- Anorexia nervosa
- Diet low in calcium
- Use of medications such as corticosteroids and anticonvulsants
- Low testosterone levels in men

- White or Asian race
- Cigarette smoking
- Excessive use of alcohol

10. What is the most effective method to prevent a postmenopausal woman from developing bone loss?

The most effective method to prevent postmenopausal bone loss is to replace estrogen. Modifying lifestyle, exercise, and vitamin supplements are important, but estrogen replacement is most effective. The use of estrogen is controversial.

11. What type of preventive measures are available for women at high risk for developing breast cancer?

There are both pharmacological and surgical interventions for the prevention of breast cancer in women at high risk for developing breast cancer. Selective estrogen receptor modulators (SERMs), such as Tamoxifen, have been shown to decrease the incidence of invasive breast cancer by 48%. These agents behave like estrogen in some tissues but block its action in others. In the breast, SERMs block estrogen, thus decreasing its ability to promote cancer. In other areas of the body, such as bone, this agent works like estrogen and promotes bone density. Surgical intervention of prophylactic total mastectomy has been shown to decrease the risk of developing breast cancer, although it is not 100% effective as a prevention measure. There is still an approximately 2% to 5% chance of developing breast cancer after a total mastectomy if microscopic cancer cells remain.

12. What are the desirable levels for total cholesterol and low-density lipoprotein (LDL) in adults to decrease the risk of coronary heart disease (CHD)?

Serum LDL and total cholesterol have a relationship in increasing the risk for developing CHD. The following table lists total cholesterol and LDL cholesterol levels and classifications according to the Third Report of the National Cholesterol Education Program.

Cholesterol Levels

Total Cholesterol (mg/dL)	LDL Cholesterol (mg/dL)
<200 Desirable	<100 Optimal
200-239 Borderline high	100-129 Above optimal
≥240 High	100-159 Borderline high
	≥190 Very high

13. **What nonlipid risk factors are associated with increased CHD risk and should be considered in prevention measures?**

Modifiable risk factors for CHD include the following:
- Hypertension
- Cigarette smoking
- Diabetes
- Obesity
- Physical inactivity
- Atherogenic diet

Maintaining blood pressure less than 140/90 mm Hg is recommended by the American Heart Association. Preventing diabetes and obesity are key factors in decreasing the risk for coronary heart disease. A diet low in fats and maintaining a healthy weight are all modifiable risk factors that patients can institute.

Nonmodifiable risk factors include the following:
- Age
- Gender (male)
- Family history of premature CHD

14. **Ms. J is a 50-year-old smoker with a family history of coronary artery disease. Her blood pressure today is 130/80 mm Hg. What guidelines will direct your treatment for her?**

The American Heart Association guidelines for prevention of heart attack and stroke include the following measures:
- No exposure to tobacco smoke
- Low-dose aspirin for people who have an increased risk for coronary heart disease
- Blood pressure maintained below 140/90 mm Hg
- Cholesterol screening every 5 years unless elevated
- At least 30 minutes of moderate-intensity physical activity preferably every day of the week

15. **A "heart-healthy" preventive health measure for adults is to limit salt intake to how many milligrams per day?**

The American Heart Association recommends that adults consume less than 6 g, or 2400 mg, of salt per day for a heart-healthy diet.

16. **According to the American Cancer Society (ACS), what breast cancer screening tests and measures should be offered to the 40-year-old woman being seen for the first time?**

According to the ACS, a 40-year-old woman should have a mammogram and clinical breast examination (CBE) by a physician or registered nurse to screen for breast cancer. The ACS also recommends monthly breast self-examination

(BSE) be done by women to detect breast changes and lumps. Other imaging tests such as magnetic resonance imaging (MRI) and ultrasound have not been proven useful for screening. MRI scans and ultrasound studies do not pick up routinely the calcifications within the breast that increase suspicion of cancer.

17. **When can women stop having Papanicolaou (Pap) tests?**

According to the ACS, Pap tests may safely be discontinued at age 70 if women have had three or more normal Pap tests in a row and no abnormal Pap tests in the last 10 years. Women who have certain risk factors such as diethylstilbestrol (DES) exposure before birth, human immunodeficiency virus (HIV) infection, a weakened immune system due to organ transplantation or chemotherapy, or long-term steroid use should continue to be screened annually if they are physically able.

18. **According to the ACS, when should Mr. S, age 45, with no family history of prostate cancer, have prostate-specific antigen (PSA) testing and a digital rectal examination for prostate cancer screening?**

Both PSA testing and digital rectal examination should be offered annually, beginning at age 50 years. High-risk groups, such as African-American men and men who have a first-degree relative diagnosed with prostate cancer at a young age, should begin testing at 45 years of age.

19. **According to the ACS Detection Guidelines, both men and women beginning at age 50 should follow what schedule of testing for colon cancer screening?**

The ACS recommends that both men and women beginning at age 50 follow one of the following testing schedules:
- Yearly fecal occult blood testing (FOBT)
- Flexible sigmoidoscopy every 5 years
- Yearly FOBT plus flexible sigmoidoscopy every 5 years (This combination is preferred over either of the two tests alone.)
- Double-contrast barium enema every 5 years
- Colonoscopy every 10 years

The virtual colonoscopy has not been approved for colon cancer screening at this time.

20. **If results for fecal occult blood are positive, which test should be recommend next?**

All positive tests for colon cancer screening, including FOBT, flexible sigmoidoscopy, and double-contrast barium enema, should be followed with a colonoscopy.

21. What lifestyle measures should be recommended to a patient to help reduce the risk of developing colon cancer?

The ACS recommends dietary preventive measures of eating 20 to 30 g of fiber a day, reducing alcohol and red meat consumption, and consuming vitamin D and calcium. Recommending that patients abstain from using tobacco is also helpful in preventing colon cancer and other types of cancers and serious diseases.

22. What is the leading cause of lung cancer in the United States?

Smoking is the number one cause of lung cancer. Smoking causes 87% of lung cancer cases. Radon is considered the second leading cause of lung cancer in the United States. Radon gas can percolate through the soil under a home or building and enter through gaps and cracks in the foundation or insulation, as well as through pipes, drains, walls, or other openings. Radon causes between 15,000 and 22,000 lung cancer deaths each year in the United States; 12% of all lung cancer deaths are linked to radon. Another leading cause of lung cancer is on-the-job exposure to cancer-causing substances or carcinogens. Asbestos is a well-known, work-related substance that can cause lung cancer, but there are many others, including uranium, arsenic, and certain petroleum products.

23. What level of sun protection factor (SPF) against ultraviolet (UV) waves should be recommended to help prevent skin cancer?

Experts recommend sunscreen products with an SPF of at least 15. The number of the SPF represents the level of sunburn protection provided by the sunscreen. SPF 4 blocks out 75% of the sun's burning UV rays, SPF 15 blocks out 93%, and SPF 30 blocks out 97% of the burning UV rays. All patients should be instructed to avoid UV waves from either the sun or tanning booths to aid in the prevention of skin cancer. Recommending that patients wear protective clothing when outdoors during the sunlight hours is another preventive measure.

24. In the clinical setting, what screening measures can be used to identify adult obesity?

The body mass index (BMI) is an indicator of body fat measured by dividing weight in kilograms (kg) by height in meters. It shows a direct relationship to morbidity and mortality in studies of large populations. In adults, obesity has been defined by the National Center for Health Statistics as a BMI greater than 27.8 for men and 27.3 for women. Anthropometric methods are measurements of skin fold thickness and the indirect assessment of body fat distribution. This technique requires training and may have lower intraobserver and interobserver reliability than BMI. The *WHR*, which is the circumference of the waist divided by the circumference of the hips, may be a better predictor of the sequelae associated with adult obesity.

25. A 26-year-old sexually active woman who has had multiple sexual partners should have what tests during her first gynecological examination?

Pap test and pelvic examination are recommended for all sexually active women and should start not later than age 21. Sexually active women, especially those who have had multiple sexual partners, should be screened for sexually transmitted diseases including chlamydia, gonorrhea, and syphilis. All sexually active women, no matter what age, who have had multiple sexual partners should be offered and counseled regarding HIV testing.

26. Which groups of patients are at risk for developing tuberculosis?

Asymptomatic persons at increased risk for developing TB include the following:
- Persons infected with HIV
- Close contacts of persons with known or suspected TB (health care workers)
- Immigrants from countries with high TB prevalence (i.e., most countries in Africa, Asia, and Latin America)
- Medically underserved, low-income populations
- Alcoholics
- Injection drug users
- Residents of long-term care facilities (e.g., prisons, nursing homes, psychiatric institutions)

27. What measures are strongly recommended by The Centers for Disease Control and Prevention (CDC) to aid in the prevention of HIV transmission?

HIV is transmitted through sexual intercourse. Either abstaining from sexual intercourse or using latex condoms or barriers during sexual intercourse is recommended. Abstaining from sharing needles or syringes with HIV-infected people and abstaining from using intravenous drugs are also recommended to prevent bloodborne transmission. HIV has been found in saliva and tears in very low quantities in some patients with acquired immunodeficiency syndrome (AIDS). Finding a small amount of HIV in a body fluid does not necessarily mean that HIV can be transmitted by that body fluid. Casual contact through closed-mouth or "social" kissing is not a risk for transmission of HIV. Because of the potential for contact with blood during "French" or open-mouth kissing, CDC recommends against engaging in this activity with a person known to be infected. However, the risk of acquiring HIV during open-mouth kissing is believed to be very low.

28. What is a contraindication for giving an influenza immunization?

Allergy to eggs. Egg proteins are used in the production of flu vaccine. If a patient has an allergy to eggs, he or she may have a severe allergic reaction to the flu shot.

29. What measures are positively shown to help prevent influenza, colds, and other respiratory viruses?

The most effective measure against influenza and infection with respiratory viruses is prevention. The flu shot has improved on the basic preventive measures such as good hygiene, handwashing, and isolating the infected persons. Even though many people believe that taking extra vitamin C and Echinacea will shorten the length of a cold, vitamin supplements have not been proven to prevent the flu, colds, or infection with other respiratory viruses.

30. According to the U.S. Preventive Services Task Force, what are the recommended guidelines for the use of pneumococcal vaccination in the prevention of pneumonia?

The pneumococcal vaccine is recommended for persons 65 years of age and older or who are otherwise at increased risk for pneumonia. High-risk groups include institutionalized persons 50 years of age or older, persons 2 years of age and older with certain medical conditions, including chronic cardiac or pulmonary disease and diabetes. Routine revaccination is not recommended, but it may be appropriate to consider revaccination in immunocompetent individuals at highest risk for morbidity and mortality from pneumococcal disease (i.e., persons 75 years of age and older or those with severe chronic disease) who were vaccinated more than 5 years previously. Revaccination with the 23-valent vaccine may be appropriate for high-risk persons who previously received the 14-valent vaccine.

31. A healthy 50-year-old man who is starting a new position is being seen for his employment physical. What vaccinations should he have received or should he receive to consider him up-to-date on vaccinations?

- Tetanus shot
- Flu shot
- Varicella and measles-mumps-rubella (MMR)

For a healthy 50-year-old, a tetanus shot should be given every 10 years, a flu shot should be given annually starting at age 50 (younger if at high risk), and both varicella and MMR should be given in adulthood if the adult was not vaccinated in childhood. Pneumonia vaccination is recommended to people age 65 and older if they are not at high risk (people with chronic diseases or who are immunocompromised).

32. For what groups of adults should a meningitis vaccination be recommended?

Adults considered at high risk for contracting meningitis include travelers to developing countries, U.S. military men and women, college students, people whose immune system does not function properly, and people with spleen problems. Meningococcal bacteria are transmitted through air droplets and by direct contact with persons already infected with the disease. The meningitis vaccine, Menomune, has been shown to provide protection against the most common strains of the disease, including serotypes A, C, Y, and W-135.

33. **An 80-year-old woman lives alone. What measures should be reviewed with her and her family to make sure she is taking precautions to prevent injuries to herself in her home?**

Most injuries in older adults occur in their homes. Reviewing safety measures with your older patients and their families will help them take measures to prevent injury. Safety measures should include adequate lighting, handrails by the tub or shower and toilet, removing area rugs, and having working smoke alarms on every level of the home.

34. **For whom should a hepatitis B vaccine be recommended?**

Adults at high risk for contracting hepatitis B are individuals with chronic liver disease, men who have sex with men, individuals who receive clotting factor products, and persons who use street drugs. This vaccine is also recommended for infants and adolescents not previously immunized. The virus is found in the blood and body fluids of infected people and can be spread through sexual contact, the sharing of needles or razors, from mother to infant during birth, and by living in a household with a chronically infected person. Safe, effective hepatitis B vaccines are available. The vaccines are used to protect everyone from newborn babies to older adults. The vaccination series, generally given as three doses over a 6-month period, protects those at risk and contributes to the elimination of this silent, highly infectious killer. The hepatitis B vaccine is recognized as the first anticancer vaccine because it can prevent liver cancer caused by hepatitis B infection.

 Key Points

- Primary goals for *Healthy People 2010* are to decrease health disparity and to increase quality and longevity of lives.
- Public health education is important in preventing spread of communicable disease.
- Cigarette smoking continues to be the leading risk factor associated with lung cancer.

 Internet Resources

The Seventh Report of the Joint National Committee on Prevention, Detection, Evaluation and Treatment of High Blood Pressure JNC 7, May 2003:
www.nhlbi.nih.gov/guidelines/hypertension

NIH, Executive Summary of the Third Report of the National Cholesterol Education Program (NCEP) Expert Panel on Detection, Evaluation, and Treatment of High Blood Cholesterol in Adults (ATP III) 2001:
www.nhlbi.nih.gov/guidelines/cholesterol

Centers for Disease Control and Prevention (HIV, STD, and TB Prevention):
www.cdc.gov/hiv/pubs/facts/transmission.htm

Bibliography

American Cancer Society. (2003). *Cancer facts and figures 2003*. Atlanta, GA: American Cancer Society.

American Cancer Society. (2003). *American Cancer Society guidelines on diet and cancer prevention.* Available at http://www.cancer.org.

American Diabetes Association. (2002). Available at http://www.diabetes.org/main/info/facts/eye/default.jsp.

American Heart Association. (2000). AHA dietary guidelines: Revision 2000, #71-0193. *Circulation, 102,* 2284-2299.

American Heart Association. (1999). AHA scientific statement: Diabetes and cardiovascular disease, #71-0175. *Circulation, 100,* 1134-1146 (Editorial in *Journal of the American College of Cardiology*).

American Heart Association. (2002). Scientific statement: AHA guidelines for primary prevention of cardiovascular disease and stroke. *Circulation, 106,* 388-391.

Freedman, A.N., et al. (2003). Estimates of the number of U.S. women who could benefit from Tamoxifen for breast cancer chemoprevention. *Journal of the National Cancer Institute, 95*(7), 526-532.

Jordan, V. C. (1998). Designer estrogens. *Scientific American,* October, 2-9.

National Cholesterol Education Program. (2001). Executive summary of the third report of the NCEP Expert Panel on Detection, Evaluation, and Treatment of High Blood and Cholesterol in Adults (adult treatment panel III). *Journal of the American Medical Association, 285,* 2486-2497.

Smith, R.A., et al. (2003). American Cancer Society guidelines for breast cancer screening: Update 2003. *CA: A Cancer Journal for Clinicians, 53,* 141-169.

U.S. Department of Health and Human Services. (2000). *Healthy People 2010: Understanding and Improving Health* (2nd ed.). Available at www.health.gov/healthypeople.

U.S. Preventive Services Task Force. (2000-2002). *Report of the U.S. Preventive Services Task Force. Guide to clinical preventive services* (2nd and 3rd ed.). Available at www.ahrq.gov/clinic/cps3dix.htm.

Section III

Challenges in Acute Care

Nutrition Support

Phyllis Ann Schiavone-Gatto and Nancy Evans-Stoner

1. **What is the incidence of protein-energy malnutrition (PEM) in the medical-surgical adult patient?**

   Protein-energy malnutrition (PEM) is a significant problem in the adult medical-surgical patient. Studies document the incidence of PEM in hospitalized medical-surgical patients as high as 40%. Malnutrition can develop as a result of acute or chronic disease processes and their treatments can result in one or all of the following: (1) decreased food intake, (2) decreased nutrient absorption, (3) increased nutrient losses, or (4) increased nutrient requirements. The presence of malnutrition can result in problems such as delayed wound healing, impaired immune function, and decreased functional status.

2. **How does one screen a patient for nutritional risk when a comprehensive nutritional evaluation is required?**

   The goal of screening is to identify the patient who needs a comprehensive nutritional assessment. It is important for nurses to use strategies to screen a patient for nutritional risk when the patient enters the health care system. Nursing admission forms can be a useful tool to complete a quick nutritional screen. The following questions are completed at the time a patient is admitted. A "yes" answer to any of the questions generates a consult to the nutritional support service for a comprehensive nutritional assessment.

   NUTRITION RISK SCREEN
   - Has unintentional weight loss exceeded 10 lb within 3 months?
   - Does the patient appear cachectic?
   - Has the patient had severe anorexia for more than 5 days?
   - Does the patient have dysphagia?
   - Has the patient had persistent vomiting for more than 3 days?
   - Has the patient had chronic diarrhea for more than 5 days?
   - Does the patient have difficulty getting adequate food?
   - Does the patient have a pressure ulcer of stage II or greater?

   Refer to the following box for a more formalized Admission Nutrition Screening Tool.

Box 14-1 Features of the Admission Nutrition Screening Tool

A. Diagnosis

If the patient has at least **ONE** of the following diagnoses, circle and proceed to section E to consider the patient **at nutritional risk** and stop here:

- Anorexia nervosa/bulimia nervosa
- Malabsorption (celiac sprue, ulcerative colitis, Crohn's disease, short bowel syndrome)
- Multiple trauma (closed head injury, penetrating trauma, multiple fractures)
- Decubitus ulcers
- Major gastrointestinal surgery within the last year
- Cachexia (temporal wasting, muscle wasting, cancer, cardiac disease)
- Coma
- Diabetes
- End-stage liver disease
- End-stage renal disease
- Nonhealing wounds

B. Nutrition Intake History

If the patient has at least **ONE** of the following symptoms, circle and proceed to section E to consider the patient **at nutritional risk** and stop here:

- Diarrhea (>500 mL for 2 days)
- Vomiting (>5 days)
- Reduced intake (less than half normal intake for more than 5 days)

C. Ideal Body Weight Standards

Compare the patient's current weight for height to the ideal body weight. If results are <80% of ideal body weight, consider the patient **at nutritional risk** and stop here.

D. Weight History

- Any recent unplanned weight loss? No _____ Yes _____ Amount (lb or kg)_____
- If yes, within the past_____ weeks or_____ months
- Current weight (lb or kg) _____
- Usual weight (lb or kg) _____
- Height (inches or cm)_____
- Find percentage of weight loss:

$$\frac{\text{Usual weight} - \text{Current weight}}{\text{Usual weight}} \times 100 = \% \text{ Weight loss}$$

- Compare the % weight loss with the chart values and circle the appropriate value.

Length of Time	Significant (%)	Severe (%)
1 week	1-2	>2
2-3 weeks	2-3	>3
1 month	4-5	>5
3 months	7-8	>8
5+ months	10	>10

- If the patient has experienced significant or severe weight loss, consider the patient **at nutritional risk**.

Box 14-1   **Features of the Admission Nutrition Screening Tool—cont'd**

E. Nurse Assessment
Using the previous criteria, what is this patient's nutritional risk?
_____ LOW NUTRITIONAL RISK
_____ AT NUTRITIONAL RISK

3. **What are components of a comprehensive nutritional assessment?**

   A comprehensive nutritional assessment includes both subjective and objective data. The goal of nutritional assessment is to identify the patient's deficits and needs. Components of a detailed nutritional assessment include the following:
   - Medical history
   - Nutritional history
   - Nutritionally focused physical examination
   - Evaluation of body weight data: % ideal body weight, % usual body weight, body mass index (BMI)
   - Serum protein status
   - Vitamin and mineral status

4. **How is malnutrition classified?**

   Malnutrition is defined as a state of overnutrition or undernutrition. Marasmus is defined as calorie malnutrition, with obvious wasting of somatic protein and fat, with preservation of visceral proteins. Kwashiorkor is protein malnutrition caused from decreased quantity or quality of protein or during periods of catabolic stress.

   EVALUATION OF BODY WEIGHT DATA
   - % Ideal body weight = Weight ÷ Ideal body weight × 100
     - 80%-90% = Mild malnutrition
     - 70%-79% = Moderate malnutrition
     - <70% = Severe malnutrition
   - % Usual body weight = Current weight ÷ Usual weight × 100
     - 85%-95% = Mild malnutrition
     - 75%-84% = Moderate malnutrition
     - <74% = Severe malnutrition

5. **What is BMI?**

   BMI is a way to define a level of obesity using the relationship between weight and height.

   $$BMI = \frac{Weight\ in\ kg}{(Height\ in\ meters) \times (Height\ in\ meters)}$$

6. How is obesity defined by BMI?

The degree of obesity based on BMI is presented in the following table.

Body Mass Index Classifications

BMI	Classification
20-25	Normal
26-29	Mild obesity
30-40	Moderate obesity
>40	Severe obesity

7. How is visceral protein status assessed?

Visceral protein status is assessed by examining serum albumin, serum trans-ferrin, and serum prealbumin. In the acute care setting, changes in these measures are often independent of nutritional status. Factors such as hydration level, liver function, and degree of catabolism affect these values. The values for normal as well as mild, moderate, and severe nutritional deficits are listed in the following table.

Values for Assessment of Visceral Protein Status

Protein	Normal	Mild	Moderate	Severe
Albumin (g/dL)	3.5-5.0	2.8-3.4	2.1-2.7	<2.1
Transferrin (mg/dL)	200-400	150-200	100-149	<100
Prealbumin (mg/dL)	16-43	10-15	5-9	<5

8. How are the energy requirements of the patient defined?

The prescription for energy needs is based on the weight goals for the patient.
- Weight maintenance: REE × 1.3, where REE = resting energy expenditure
- Weight gain: REE × 1.5
- Weight reduction: REE × 1.0, not below 800 nonprotein kcal/day

The REE is calculated through a predictive equation and then is adjusted for activity/stress level to estimate the total energy expenditure (TEE). There are a number of equations available to predict the REE; the most reliable in nonobese and obese individuals is the Mifflin-St. Jeor equation:

$$\text{REE (females)} = 9.99 \times \text{Weight (kg)} + 6.25 \times \text{Height (cm)} - 4.92 \times \text{Age (yr)} - 161$$
$$\text{REE (males)} = 9.99 \times \text{Weight (kg)} + 6.25 \times \text{Height (cm)} - 4.92 \times \text{Age (yr)} + 5$$

9. **How is energy expenditure measured?**

Energy expenditure can be measured by indirect calorimetry. Portable carts as well as handheld devices are available to measure the oxygen consumed and the carbon dioxide produced in order to calculate the REE. To ensure the greatest reliability, these measurements should be obtained from clinicians who are skilled with administering the test. Measured energy expenditure is most useful in stressed patients or in patients whose condition is unstable.

10. **How are protein requirements determined?**
   - Normal needs
   - Needs in stress

11. **How does one select the type of enteral access device to provide nutritional supplementation?**
   - Length of time feeding is requires
   - Prepyloric and postpyloric feeding and prevention of aspiration
   - Gastrointestinal (GI) problem and anatomical considerations

12. **What are the factors that should be considered in selecting the appropriate type of enteral formula?**
   - Gastrointestinal function
   - Nutritional requirements
   - Disease process
   - Enteral access device
   - Cost

13. **What is the difference between total parenteral nutrition (TPN) and peripheral parenteral nutrition (PPN)?**

The nutritional components of PPN are similar to those of TPN but have a lower concentration so it can be delivered by the peripheral veins. The dextrose concentration is 5% to 10% and the amino acids are 3% concentration. It can be used in patients with mild or moderate malnutrition to provide partial or total nutrition support when they are not able to ingest adequate calories orally or enterally or when central venous access is not feasible. Typically, PPN can be used for short periods (up to 2 weeks) because tolerance is limited and peripheral veins are limited.

TPN has a high glucose concentration, usually 15% to 25%, along with electrolytes and amino acids. It provides a hyperosmolar formulation (1300 to 1800 mOsm/L) that must be delivered by a large vein, usually the superior vena cava. TPN can be administered for weeks to years for patients who require long-term management.

14. **How are blood glucose levels managed in patients receiving TPN?**

When first initiating TPN, the blood glucose levels are checked 4 hours into the infusion to assess tolerance to glucose load. When the TPN is cycled over 12 hours in preparation for home administration, glucose levels are checked before starting TPN, then 1 to 2 hours into the TPN infusion, and then 1 to 2 hours after the TPN infusion is completed. Based on these values, the patient may or may not require insulin administration subcutaneously. If the patient requires insulin on a sliding scale, then two thirds of the sliding scale insulin can be added to the TPN bag.

15. **What are the advantages of feeding the patient enterally rather than with TPN?**

In many settings, enteral tube feedings have been proven to be safer and more cost effective than parenteral feeding. Studies have shown that there are fewer infectious complications in patients fed enterally following trauma. Intestinal function is preserved by using enteral tube feedings rather than parenteral nutrition in patients with head injury.

16. **What are the proper administration techniques for the safe delivery of enteral therapy?**

Enteral administration depends on the type of tube being used. It can be delivered by continuous or intermittent administration. Continuous feedings are used when a controlled amount of formula needs to be delivered via the enteral feeding tube in order to preserve GI tolerance. This kind of feeding can minimize the risk of aspiration from reflux from a high residual volume or from a weakened lower esophageal sphincter. Continuous feedings are used for feeding into the small intestine. They can be initiated in an adult whose condition is stable at 30 mL/hr and advanced by 10 to 20 mL/hr every 4 to 6 hours until the goal rate is achieved.

Intermittent or bolus feedings are delivered by gravity using a bag or syringe set up. Gravity feedings are used for patients who are medically stable and when a large volume of low viscosity enteral feeding formula is needed, when the diameter of the feeding tube is wide, and when the patient has adequate absorptive capacity to tolerate inconsistent formula flow. The gravity feeding bags are used and the formula is administered intermittently for 20- to 30-minute periods throughout the day. Some of the feeding delivery sets have roller clamps to control the flow rate of the gravity feeding.

17. **Does the enteral formula provide adequate fluid to maintain hydration status?**

No, it does not provide adequate fluid to maintain hydration status. The patient must flush with water with a syringe throughout the 24-hour period to ensure hydration if he or she cannot take fluids by mouth. To ensure that adequate hydration is obtained, calculate the total volume of the tube feed and multiply that number by the percent of free water in formula. Then multiply 35 mL by body weight in kilograms. Subtract the first number from the second number to give the number of milliliters needed for hydration.

18. **What are the nursing strategies for monitoring and preventing a tube feeding–related aspiration?**

Tube feeding aspiration is a serious complication that can lead to pneumonia. Traditionally, blue dye has been added to the formulas, and tracheal secretions were monitored for the presence of blue discoloration indicating the occurrence of aspiration. This practice is now contraindicated due to systemic absorption of the blue dye. The following procedure instructs how to prevent aspiration of enteral tube feedings.
- Keep the head of the bed elevated approximately 30 to 45 degrees while tube feeding is being administered and then for 1 hour after feeding has been completed.
- Check residual volumes before administering the next feeding.
  - If more than 200 mL are withdrawn, recheck in 2 hours.
  - If the volume is still high after 2 hours, the feeding tube may need to be placed at the ligament of Treitz.

19. **What are the most common GI problems related to enteral feedings?**
- Abdominal pain
- Abdominal distention
- Nausea
- Diarrhea

These are all signs of intolerance to feedings. Approximately 20% of patients who receive enteral feedings report nausea and vomiting. Vomiting does increase the risk of aspiration, pneumonia, and sepsis. The nausea and vomiting etiology is usually multifactorial and is usually seen in patients with delayed gastric emptying. This can occur from hypotension, sepsis, or stress, or it may follow anesthesia and surgery. Many medications reduce gastric motility. Diarrhea may be related to the osmolarity.

20. **If delayed gastric emptying in a patient receiving enteral feedings is suspected, how should it be managed?**
- Reduce or discontinue narcotic use.
- Switch to low-fat formula.
- Administer formula at room temperature.
- Decrease the infusion rate by 20 to 25 mL/hr.
- Consider adding a prokinetic agent, such as metoclopramide.

21. **How should diarrhea be managed in the patient receiving enteral feedings?**

If diarrhea is clinically significant, start Kaopectate, which does not alter the motility of the bowel, and obtain a stool culture for *Clostridium difficile*. If the culture is negative, consider an enteral formula with added fiber, change the formula, or use an antidiarrhea agent (loperamide, diphenoxylate, paregoric, or octreotide).

22. What are the most common mechanical complications of an enteral feeding tube?

The following are the most common mechanical complications of enteral feeding:
- The *placement* of the tube can cause bleeding, tracheal or parenchymal perforation, GI tract perforation leading to abscess formation and peritonitis, increased intracranial pressure, and respiratory complications.
- The *characteristics of the feeding tube* can cause sinusitis, dental problems, pneumonia, aggravation of esophageal varices, cellulitis, necrotizing fasciitis, fistulas, and wound.
- *Tube clogging* is a primary problem with tube feeding. Most of the clogging can be prevented by frequent flushing of the tube before and after medication administration and formula infusion. Some declogging methods include warm water or sodium bicarbonate/pancrelipase mixture.
- *Aspiration* is a serious complication and can be life threatening in malnourished patients. Aspiration symptoms are dyspnea, tachypnea, wheezing, rales, tachycardia, anxiety, agitation, and cyanosis. Prevention includes raising the head of the bed to 30 to 45 degrees during feeding administration and for 1 hour after and checking residual volumes. An assessment of residual volume should be done on a schedule, with adjustment of feedings as indicated.
- *Infection* can be minimized by careful attention when tubes are placed.

23. What is refeeding syndrome?

Refeeding syndrome is defined as the metabolic and physiological consequences of depletion, repletion, compartmental shifts, and interrelationships of phosphorus, potassium, magnesium, glucose metabolism, vitamin deficiency, and fluid resuscitation.

The sole cause of the metabolic response to refeeding is the shift from body fat and conversion to carbohydrates during a period of relative or actual starvation. This causes the serum insulin levels to rise, thus causing intracellular movement of electrolytes for the use of metabolic pathways. There can be a drop below the normal levels of serum magnesium, potassium, and phosphorus. There is a rise in the insulin production, which antagonizes the action of glucagons in the liver, inhibits fatty acid mobilization, and reduces glycogenolysis and gluconeogenesis, leading to low serum glucose levels and other complications.

24. Which patients are at risk for refeeding syndrome?

- Classic kwashiorkor
- Marasmus

- Anorexia nervosa
- Chronic alcoholism
- Chronic malnutrition
- Morbid obesity with massive weight loss
- Prolonged intravenous hydration
- Prolonged fasting or NPO (nothing by mouth) status for 7 to 10 days
- Significant stress

25. How is refeeding syndrome managed?

Electrolyte abnormalities need to be corrected before starting nutrition support. The nutrition support rule of thumb is to start low and go slow with increases, regardless of the route. Electrolytes, fluid balance, and metabolic response must be monitored closely once the nutrition support has begun. This should help reduce the hyperinsulinemia, intracellular electrolyte transport, and clinical symptoms of refeeding. Also, give the appropriate vitamin supplementation and avoid overfeeding.

26. What key nutritional parameters should be monitored in the patient receiving parenteral or enteral nutrition?

- Electrolytes
- Weight
- Transport proteins

27. How is a patient readied for discharge to home on TPN or total enteral nutrition (TEN)?

The TPN/TEN should be cycled to a 12-hour infusion in preparation for home. The TPN can be cycled from 24 hours to 16 hours in a diabetic patient and then, when the patient's condition is stable, to a 12-hour infusion. Finger-stick blood glucose should be check before starting TPN, 1 to 2 hours into the infusion and then again 1 to 2 hours after the infusion is completed. If the finger-stick blood glucose is elevated, then a glucose monitor should be ordered for the patient and teaching should begin. If the patient requires insulin subcutaneously or added to the TPN solution, diabetic teaching should begin in preparation for discharge to home. The patient will then need a prescription for insulin, syringes, lancets, strips, and a sliding scale.

TEN can be advanced to a 24-hour goal and then cycled to a 12-hour cycle by increasing the rate as previously mentioned.

Develop a collaborative relationship with the discharge planning nurse. The nurse gives the information on the infusion company that will be used for the patient. Also, identify an attending physician who will manage the TPN at home.

28. Are nutritional therapies delivered in the home setting covered by most insurance providers?

Coverage for nutritional therapies such as TPN and TEN varies based on the specific insurance provider. Administering specialized nutrition at home is costly: TPN can cost approximately $300 per day and TEN can cost $40 to $60 per day.

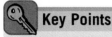 **Key Points**

- Nutritional assessment is a critical component in the comprehensive care of adult patients in the acute care setting. All patients should be screened for risk and those at risk should have a comprehensive nutritional assessment.
- TPN and TEN are complementary therapies that support the patient who is unable to meet their nutritional needs with oral intake. Both therapies should be individualized to the goals for calories and protein.
- Nutritional support is not without potential complication. Routine reassessment must occur to evaluate the patient's response to therapy.

 Internet Resources

Nutrition.org (American Society for Nutritional Sciences):
www.nutrition.org

Food and Nutrition Information Center:
www.nal.usda.gov/fnic

Nutrition.Gov (Online Federal Government Information on Nutrition):
www.nutrition.gov

Bibliography

Attar, A., & Messing, B. (2001). Evidence-based prevention of catheter infection during parenteral nutrition. *Current Opinion in Clinical Nutrition and Metabolic Care, 4*,211-218.

Evans-Stoner, N., Cantwell, C., & Compher, C. (2005). Management of clients with malnutrition. In J.M. Black & J. Hokanson Hawks (Eds.), *Medical-surgical nursing: Clinical management for positive outcomes* (7th ed.). St. Louis: Mosby.

Lord, L.M. (2003). Restoring and maintaining patency of enteral feeding tubes. *Nutrition in Clinical Practice, 18*, 422-425.

Parrish, C. (2003). Enteral feeding: The art and the science. *Nutrition in Clinical Practice, 18*(1), 76-83.

Robinson, M.K., et al. (2003). Improving nutritional screening of hospitalized patients: The role of pre-albumin. *Journal of Parenteral and Enteral Nutrition, 27*(6), 389-395.

Rolandelli, R., et al. (Eds.). (2004). *Clinical nutrition: Enteral and tube feeding* (4th ed.). Philadelphia: W.B. Saunders.

Shils M.E., et al. (Eds.). (1999). *Modern nutrition in health and disease* (9th ed.). Baltimore: Williams & Wilkins.

Speerhas, R., et al. (2003). Maintaining normal blood glucose concentrations with TPN: Is it necessary to taper TN? *Nutrition in Clinical Practice, 18*(5), 414-416.

Chapter 15

Traumatic Injuries

Corinna P. Sicoutris

1. **Describe the differences between a trauma primary, secondary, and tertiary survey.**

   Evaluation of a trauma patient should be comprehensive, systematic, and prioritized. In the primary survey, life-threatening injuries are identified and treated. The ABCDEs, similar to the ABCs of basic life support, refer to the sequential method of initially and simultaneously assessing and managing a trauma patient in the resuscitation bay.

   A: Airway with C-spine control
   B: Breathing and ventilation
   C: Circulation with hemorrhage control
   D: Disability/neurological status
   E: Exposure and environmental control

   The secondary survey begins only after the primary survey is completed, resuscitation is underway, and hemodynamic stability is restored. It is a systematic head-to-toe assessment, including both a history and a physical. The objective is to carefully examine all regions of the body to identify injuries.

   The tertiary survey takes place after the primary and secondary surveys are completed, often 24 hours into the hospital stay of noncritical trauma patients and potentially much longer for a patient admitted to the intensive care unit. It is a thorough head to toe physical assessment performed to identify any delayed or missed diagnoses. It should be done before the patient ambulates when it is thought that the patient can participate in the physical examination.

2. **Which cranial nerve (CN) is responsible for the appearance of the "blown pupil?"**

   CN III, the oculomotor nerve, runs just beneath the tentorium and has parasympathetic fibers that run along the length of the surface. When there is increased pressure in the cranial vault to the extent that pressure is transmitted downward onto the tentorium, as in the case of uncal herniation, the parasympathetic fibers are unable to respond to the normal sympathetic response of pupillary dilation. This inability and in extreme case paralysis of the parasympathetic fibers make the oculomotor nerve unable to constrict the pupils and the appearance of "blown pupils" is observed.

3. **Is it appropriate to use antibiotics to treat a cerebrospinal fluid (CSF) leak resulting from a basilar skull fracture?**

No. CSF otorrhea or rhinorrhea resulting from a basilar skull fracture should not be treated prophylactically with antibiotics. The main concern with a CSF leak is meningitis. However, the use of prophylactic antibiotics may allow a more resistant organism to grow, thereby making it more difficult to treat and increasing morbidity. Management of a CSF leak is performed by elevating the head of the bed to 60 degrees and considering placement of a lumbar drain.

4. **What is the dosing regimen of steroids recommended to treat patients following a blunt spinal cord injury (SCI)?**

Methylprednisolone is a glucocorticoid used to improve neurological recovery following an acute SCI. The high-dose steroid should be administered within the first 8 hours of injury in patients with nonpenetrating, incomplete SCI. The initial loading dose is 30 mg/kg over 15 minutes in the first hour, followed by 5.4 mg/kg/hr as a continuous infusion for the next 23 hours.

5. **Compare the chest radiograph findings of a pneumothorax, a hemothorax, an occult pneumothorax, and a tension pneumothorax.**

Chest Radiograph Findings of a Pneumothorax, Hemothorax, Occult Pneumothorax, and Tension Pneumothorax

Chest Radiograph Findings	Radiographic Appearance
Pneumothorax	Thin white line representing the visceral parietal pleura and absence of lung markings above that line giving the appearance of a hyperlucent area
Hemothorax	Unilateral opacification and complete "white out"
Occult pneumothorax	Not appreciated on chest radiograph, but may be detected on a thoracic or abdominal computed tomography scan
Tension pneumothorax	No radiographic findings

6. **How is tension pneumothorax treated?**

It is treated with immediate needle decompression using a large-bore needle inserted between the second and third intercostal space along the midclavicular line.

7. **Describe the radiograph findings suggestive of a blunt aortic injury.**

Traumatic rupture of the aorta is a tear in the wall of the aorta generally caused by a rapid deceleration injury. Most patients die at the scene. Those who survive to the hospital generally are hypotensive but respond, at least initially, to fluid therapy. On chest radiograph, the following signs should increase your suspicion of a blunt aortic injury:

- Widened mediastinum (>8 cm)
- Loss of aortic knob
- Apical cap
- Large hemothorax or pleural effusion
- Deviation of the trachea to the right
- Deviation of the esophagus to the right (nasogastric tube deviation)
- Concomitant injuries (first 3 rib fractures, sternal fracture, scapula fracture)
- Elevation and rightward shift of mainstem bronchus
- Loss of aortopulmonary window

No radiographic finding alone is diagnostic for a blunt aortic injury but a widened mediastinum is the most consistent finding and should always raise your index of suspicion. In the presence of these radiographic signs, further evaluation using computed tomography (CT) or aortography is indicated.

8. **What is Beck's triad?**

Beck's triad is the classic triad of signs suggestive of cardiac tamponade and includes hypotension, jugular venous distention (JVD), and muffled heart sounds.

Cardiac tamponade may be a result of either penetrating or blunt trauma and may be caused by as little as 75 mL of blood in the pericardial sac. It should be considered in patients with hypotension out of proportion to obvious blood loss coupled with a high index of suspicion based on the mechanism of injury. Other signs of cardiac tamponade include hemodynamic instability, equalization of filling pressures, pulsus paradoxus (decreasing of systolic pressure on inspiration), cyanosis, exsanguinating hemothorax (if associated with pericardial tear), and Kussmaul's sign (increase in central venous pressure on inspiration in a spontaneously breathing patient).

9. **Is there an elevation of cardiac isoenzymes in a patient suffering from a blunt cardiac injury (BCI)?**

No. BCI represents a spectrum of injury ranging from asymptomatic dysrhythmias to frank cardiac rupture. Cardiac enzymes do not correlate with the presence of, severity of, or complications associated with BCI. Diagnosis of BCI is made using a screening electrocardiogram and a transthoracic echocardiogram (TTE). A transesophageal (TEE) echocardiogram may be used if the TTE is inadequate.

10. **What are the clinical manifestations of a pelvic fracture?**

Awake patients may complain of pelvic pain and an inability to void, particularly in the presence of an associated urethral disruption. On examination, stability of the pelvis can be ascertained by performing manual anteroposterior (AP) and lateral compression and the rocking maneuver. Inspection of the perineum, scrotum, external female genitalia, vagina, and rectum is essential to identify soft tissue injuries or lacerations resulting in an open pelvic fracture. A neurosensory evaluation including sphincter tone, perineal sensation, and lower extremity function should also be performed to identify a neurological injury.

11. When is diagnostic peritoneal lavage (DPL) considered positive?

A DPL is positive when more than 100,000 red blood cells (RBCs), more than 50,000 white blood cells (WBCs), bile, bacteria, or food particles are found.

12. Is hypotension an early symptom of hemorrhagic shock?

No. Hemorrhagic shock is the most common form of shock in trauma patients and hypotension occurs after 30% to 40% of the body's blood volume has been lost. Therefore, when hypotension is observed in a trauma patient, the patient is in class III shock. The following table lists the symptoms of hemorrhagic shock.

Classification of Hemorrhagic Shock

	Class I	Class II	Class III	Class IV
Blood loss (mL)	Up to 750	750-1500	1500-2000	>2000
Blood loss (% blood volume)	Up to 15%	15%-30%	30%-40%	>40%
Heart rate (beats/min)	<100	>100	>120	>140
Blood pressure (mm Hg)	Normal	Normal	↓	↓
Pulse pressure	Normal or ↑	↓	↓	↓
Respiratory rate (per min)	14-20	20-30	30-40	>35
Urine output (mL/hr)	>30	20-30	5-15	Negligible
Mental status	Slightly anxious	Mildly anxious	Anxious and confused	Confused lethargic

13. What is the diagnostic test of choice for a motor vehicle accident patient who has blood at the urethral meatus?

A retrograde urethrogram is performed by placing a urinary catheter into the urethra and gently injecting contrast. Three-view cystograms are then shot with the catheter in place to assess the cause of the hematuria.

14. Describe both the hard signs and the soft signs of an arterial injury. How are they different from venous injuries?

The three components of the neurovascular assessment of an extremity are (1) vascular examination, (2) neurological examination, and (3) soft tissue and skeletal examination. These elements, plus a detailed history of mechanism of injury, prehospital blood loss, and history of pulse examinations, allow one to assess the potential for vascular injury.

The hard signs of an arterial injury are as follows:
- Absent or diminished pulses
- Distal ischemia (pain, pallor, poikilothermia, paresthesia, paralysis)
- Expanding or pulsatile hematoma
- Pulsatile bleeding
- Palpable bruit or thrill

Hard signs of arterial injury are clear indications for surgical exploration and repair. Soft signs of arterial injury include the following:
- Small, nonpulsatile hematoma
- Proximity of penetrating wound or blunt injury to the artery
- Neurological deficit in the affected extremity
- History of arterial bleeding

Soft signs of arterial injury can be further evaluated with angiography, non-invasive vascular studies (e.g., ankle brachial index [ABI], duplex studies), or serial physical examinations.

Signs of venous injuries are swelling, hemorrhage, or venous engorgement. Venous injuries typically are either repaired or ligated in the operating room.

15. What is the "trauma triad of death"?

The trauma triad of death refers to three lethal complications in the resuscitation of trauma patients:
- Metabolic acidosis
- Coagulopathy
- Hypothermia

16. Describe the phases of the surgical technique of damage control.

Phase	Intervention
I	Initial laparotomy is done for hemorrhage control, contamination containment, and intra-abdominal packing.
II	Continued resuscitation is done in the intensive care unit with the goal of optimizing hemodynamics and perfusion, and of correcting acidosis, hypothermia, and coagulopathies. Monitor for intra-abdominal hypertension and provide ventilatory support.
III	Re-exploration is done for removal of packing, definitive repair of intra-abdominal injuries, and closure if possible.

Phases of the Surgical Technique of Damage Control

17. What is the difference between intra-abdominal hypertension (IAH) and abdominal compartment syndrome (ACS)?

IAH is an elevation of intra-abdominal pressure that is typically measured in the bladder using a Foley catheter, sterile saline, and an arterial line pressure transducer zeroed at the symphysis pubis. ACS, on the other hand, is a clinical syndrome evidenced by the presence of IAH as well as any number of the following physical findings or clinical effects:
- Firm, distended abdomen
- Elevated peak airway pressures (>40 cm H_2O)
- Decreased thoracic compliance
- Elevated filling pressures
- Oliguria
- Elevated intracranial pressure
- Abdominal wall ischemia

ACS can be primary, resulting from ongoing bleeding following laparotomy, or secondary, developing in patients without intra-abdominal injury after an aggressive fluid resuscitation for massive trauma.

18. What intra-abdominal injuries are commonly missed on a CT scan?
- Hollow viscus injuries
- Pancreatic injuries
- Diaphragmatic injuries

19. Is a focused assessment by sonography in trauma (FAST) examination better at diagnosing injuries commonly missed on CT scan?

No. FAST examination is a noninvasive method of assessing hemoperitoneum in the trauma resuscitation area. In general, it is less sensitive than CT in diagnosing hemoperitoneum, and it is significantly less sensitive than CT in identifying solid organ injury. A FAST examination is performed by a trained member of the trauma team and consists of four views: subxiphoid, Morison's pouch, splenorenal recess, and the pelvis.

20. Which vaccines are given to a trauma patient following a splenectomy?

Patients who have undergone a splenectomy are at risk for developing overwhelming postsplenectomy infection (OPSI). The organisms most commonly responsible for OPSI are *Haemophilus influenzae, Meningococcus, Streptococcus pneumoniae, Escherichia coli,* and *Staphylococcus aureus.* Following a splenectomy, patients should receive Pneumovax, influenza, and meningococcal vaccines. They should also inform their primary care practitioner of their asplenic state and receive prophylactic antibiotics before undergoing any invasive procedures, such as dental work.

21. **What is the "3 for 1" rule referred to in the initial fluid resuscitation of trauma patients?**

According to the *Advanced Trauma Life Support for Doctors* (American College of Surgeons, 1997), the "3 for 1" rule states that for every 1 mL of blood lost, 3 mL of volume should be replaced. For class I and class II shock, crystalloid solutions are typically administered. In class III and class IV shock, blood replacement may also be necessary. For example, if a trauma patient is estimated to have lost 500 mL of blood volume, he or she would require at least 1500 mL of volume replacement. However, this is a guideline, which, when taken out of context of a specific clinical scenario, could result in either overresuscitation or underresuscitation of trauma patients. The key to measuring fluid resuscitation in a trauma patient is to monitor the response to volume as well as to measure end-organ perfusion, such as measuring urine output.

22. **How does one calculate fluid requirements in a burn patient using the Parkland formula?**

The Parkland formula is used to guide the volume of crystalloid resuscitation that should occur over the first 24 hours after burn injury. The formula is 4 mL/kg per percentage of body surface area (BSA). The BSA is calculated using the rule of nines, taking into account only second- and third-degree burns. Once calculated, administer one half of the total volume over the first 8 hours and the second half over the following 16 hours. The first 8 hours begins at the time of the burn, not at the time of presentation to the hospital. The guide to the adequacy of the fluid resuscitation of burn patients is urine output at a minimum rate of 0.5 mL/kg/hr.

EXAMPLE: A 60-kg woman suffers burns over 40% of her BSA. Her total fluid requirement, based on the Parkland formula, for the first 24 hours is 9600 mL of crystalloid. She should receive 4800 mL within the first 8 hours after the burn injury, followed by 4800 mL over the next 16 hours.

23. **What are the risk factors for the development of deep vein thrombosis (DVT) in trauma patients?**

DVT poses a significant risk to trauma patients, with incidence thought to be as high as 65% in untreated trauma patients. DVT is not only a major cause of morbidity but also mortality with pulmonary embolisms (PEs) being responsible for as many as 200,000 deaths per year. Virchow's triad of venous stasis, endothelial damage, and hypercoagulability has been described as being responsible for the development of venous thromboembolic complications in trauma patients. In general, trauma patients are at increased risk for development of DVTs because of immobilization, direct venous trauma, skeletal trauma, multiple transfusions, and severity of injuries.

To provide the most appropriate and cost-effective prophylaxis, risk can be stratified into the categories listed in the following table.

Risk Categories for Deep Vein Thrombosis

Low Risk	High Risk	Very High Risk
Age >40 yr	Age >50 yr	Spinal cord injury (SCI)
ISS >9	ISS ≥16	AIS—Head/neck ≥3 + long bone fracture (upper or lower)
Blood transfusion	Femoral central venous catheter in trauma resuscitation	Severe pelvic fracture (posterior element) + long bone fracture (upper or lower)
Surgical procedure ≥2 hr	AIS ≥3 (any body region)	Multiple (≥3) long bone fractures
Lower extremity fracture	GCS ≤8	
Pelvis fracture	SCI	
SCI	Pelvis fracture	
Immobilization	Femur or tibia fracture	
Pregnancy	Venous injury	
Estrogen therapy		
History of deep vein thrombosis or pulmonary embolus		
Malignancy		
Hypercoagulable state		
Extensive soft tissue trauma		
Heart failure		

AIS, Abbreviated injury scale; *GCS*, Glasgow Coma Score; *ISS*, Injury Severity Score.

24. **Which fractures are most commonly associated with compartment syndrome?**
   - Closed tibia fractures
   - Supracondylar humerus fractures

25. **What is compartment syndrome?**

   Compartment syndrome occurs when pressure increases within a fixed space to a point where perfusion becomes impaired. One should have a high index of suspicion when passive stretching is limited and painful following trauma.

   The following are manifestations of compartment syndrome:
   - Severe pain
   - Paresthesias (late finding)
   - Swollen compartment
   - Pain on passive stretch

- Sensory deficits
- Pulse change (late finding) or loss of motor function (may be earliest sign)

The extent of damage is a result of the degree of elevation of compartment pressures as well as the duration of the pressure elevation. In general, compartment syndrome can be caused by any injury that produces tissue edema.

26. **Describe the zones of injury in the neck.**

    Injury to the neck can be either blunt or penetrating in nature. In both cases, the neck is broken down into three anatomical zones:
    - *Zone I:* Area between the clavicle and the cricoid cartilage
      - Potential injuries: Subclavian, innominate vein, common carotid artery, vertebral arteries, lung, trachea, esophagus, spinal cord, thoracic duct, cervical nerve roots
    - *Zone II:* Area between the cricoid cartilage and angle of the mandible
      - Potential injuries: Vertebral arteries, carotid sheath, jugular veins, esophagus, trachea, spinal cord, larynx
    - *Zone III:* Area between the angle of the mandible and the skull base
      - Potential injuries: Pharynx, jugular veins, vertebral arteries, internal carotid arteries, CN XII (hypoglossal), intracranial injury

27. **Compare and contrast an epidural hematoma (EDH), a subdural hematoma (SDH), a subarachnoid hemorrhage (SAH), a cerebral contusion, and a diffuse axonal injury (DAI).**

Comparison of Epidural Hematoma, Subdural Hematoma, Subarachnoid Hemorrhage, Cerebral Contusion, and Diffuse Axonal Injury

Type of Head Injury	Location	Cause	Presentation
Epidural hematoma (EDH)	Epidural space, between the skull and dura mater	Result of trauma to the middle meningeal artery caused by a skull fracture. Venous bleeding secondary to skull fractures in the temporal or temporoparietal region.	Lucid interval, when the patient is awake and communicative and then a rapid neurological deterioration. Head computed tomography (CT) scan may have a biconvex or lenticular appearance.
Subdural hematoma (SDH)	Subdural space between the dura and arachnoid matter	Tearing of the bridging veins between the cerebral cortex and draining venous sinus.	Head CT scan has concave or crescent appearance and may layer along the surface of the hemisphere.

Continued

Comparison of Epidural Hematoma, Subdural Hematoma, Subarachnoid Hemorrhage, Cerebral Contusion, and Diffuse Axonal Injury—cont'd			
Type of Head Injury	**Location**	**Cause**	**Presentation**
Subarachnoid hemorrhage (SAH)	Sulci and basilar cisterns	Head trauma.	
Cerebral contusions	Frontal or temporal lobes	Usually seen in conjunction with subdural hematomas.	
Diffuse axonal injury (DAI)		Acceleration-deceleration mechanism.	Focal hemorrhages best seen on magnetic resonance imaging.

28. **Is radiographic imaging of the spine adequate to clear spine injury in trauma patients?**

    No. Every trauma patient with an appropriate mechanism of injury should be suspected of having a spinal column injury until proven otherwise. Spines must be evaluated both for the potential for bony injury as well as soft tissue and ligamentous injury.

    CERVICAL SPINE CLEARANCE
    - Reliable clinical examination (when possible), assessing for pain, swelling, step-off, deformity, and range of motion
    - Three views on plain radiograph: odontoid, lateral, and AP (must visualize C1-T1)
    - If unable to perform any part of the examination, maintain cervical immobilization with a collar
    - May do CT of the neck to look for bony injury or to better visualize vertebrae not seen well on plain films
    - May use magnetic resonance imaging (MRI) to assess for soft tissue or ligamentous injury as well as injury to the spinal cord
    - May use flexion-extension films

    THORACIC AND LUMBAR SPINE CLEARANCE
    - Reliable clinical examination (when possible), assessing for pain, swelling, step-off, or deformity
    - Two views on plain radiograph: AP and lateral
    - May use oblique views
    - May use CT of the thoracic and lumbar spine to look for bony injury or to better visualize vertebrae not seen well on plain films
    - May use MRI to assess for soft tissue or ligamentous injury as well as injury to the spinal cord

29. **What is the most commonly injured organ in penetrating trauma?**

The small bowel is the most commonly injured organ in the abdominal cavity because it occupies most of the peritoneum, thereby exposing itself to injury. Also, because it is attached to the mesentery, it is mobile and can occupy almost any part of the peritoneal cavity, depending on patient position and trajectory.

Diagnosing a small bowel injury on a CT scan can be challenging, particularly in the early stages. Some of the CT findings may be free fluid without evidence of solid organ injury, mesenteric infiltration, free intraperitoneal air, or bowel wall thickness.

30. **What are the urgent indications for a laparotomy in a trauma patient?**
    - Hemodynamic instability
    - Peritoneal findings
    - Anterior penetrating wounds below the fifth intercostal line
    - Free air
    - Bullets below the diaphragm on radiograph

31. **Describe the grades of injury for the liver.**

The liver is the most commonly injured intra-abdominal organ. Management of liver injuries has and continues to evolve. Grades of liver injury are shown in the following table.

Grades of Liver Injury

Grade	Type of Injury	Description
I	Hematoma	Subcapsular, <10% surface area
	Laceration	Capsular tear, <1 cm parenchymal depth
II	Hematoma	Subcapsular, 10% to 50% surface area
		Intraparenchymal, <10 cm in diameter
	Laceration	Capsular tear, 1 to 3 cm parenchymal depth, <10 cm in length
III	Hematoma	Subcapsular, >50% surface area or expanding
		Ruptured subcapsular or parenchymal hematoma
		Intraparenchymal hematoma, >10 cm and expanding
	Laceration	Parenchymal depth, >3 cm
IV	Laceration	Parenchymal disruption involving 25% to 75% hepatic lobe or 1 to 3 Couinaud's segments
V	Laceration	Parenchymal disruption, >75% of hepatic lobe or >3 Couinaud's segments within a single lobe
	Vascular	Juxtahepatic venous injuries
VI	Vascular	Hepatic avulsion

32. What are the indications for tetanus prophylaxis?

Tetanus (lockjaw) is both preventable and lethal. It is caused by *Clostridium tetani* and is a spore-producing anaerobic bacillus, which releases an endotoxin, called tetanospasmin, which acts on the central nervous system. Its incubation period can be as long as 21 days. Patients who have sustained open fractures, deep (>1 cm) wounds, abrasions, or lacerations, have signs of contamination or devitalized tissue, or have evidence of infection or ischemia all should receive active immunization against tetanus.

33. What is the most common cause of trauma in older adults?

Falls are the greatest cause of trauma in people older than 75 years of age and the second leading cause of trauma in people between 65 and 74 years of age. When evaluating an older trauma patient who has fallen, it is essential to carefully investigate not only the injuries sustained during the fall, but also the reason for the fall. Common reasons for falls in older adults are impaired mobilization, instability, altered gait, motor/sensory deficits, syncope, cardiac dysrhythmias, anemia, cerebral ischemia, and hypoglycemia. A relatively minor fall can have functionally devastating and lasting effects in older adults.

Key Points

- Trauma is a national public health problem and is responsible for significant cost, disability, and mortality across all age-groups.
- Prompt recognition and management of injuries is essential.
- The organization of a multidisciplinary trauma team within a designated trauma system who has access to resources is of paramount importance in the diagnosis of injury and management of these complex cases.

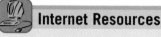

Internet Resources

Trauma.Org:
www.trauma.org

Trauma.Org (Trauma Moulage Scenarios):
www.trauma.org/resus/moulage/moulage.html

American Trauma Society:
www.amtrauma.org

Bibliography

Allen, T.L., et al. (2004). Computed tomographic scanning without oral contrast solution for blunt bowel and mesenteric injuries in abdominal trauma. *Journal of Trauma, 56*(2), 314-322.

American College of Surgeons: Committee on Trauma. (1997). *Advanced trauma life support for doctors* (6th ed.). Chicago: Author.

Cartotto, R.C., et al. (2002). How well does the Parkland formula estimate actual fluid resuscitation volumes? *Journal of Burn Care and Rehabilitation, 23*(4), 258-265.

Cera, S.M., et al. (2003). Physiologic predictors of survival in post-traumatic arrest. *The American Surgeon 69*(2), 140-144.

Haskell, R.M. Trauma. In P. Logan (Ed.). (1999). *Principles of practice for the acute care nurse practitioner* (pp. 347-419). Stamford, CT: Appleton & Lange.

Mattox, K.L., Feliciano, D.V., & Moore, E.E. (Eds.). (2000). *Trauma* (4th ed.). New York: McGraw-Hill.

Peitzman, A.B., et al. (Eds.). (2002). *The trauma manual* (2nd ed.). Philadelphia: Lippincott Williams & Wilkins.

Schwartz-Arad, D., Levin, L., & Ashkenazi, M. (2004). Treatment options of untreatable traumatized anterior maxillary teeth for future use of dental implantation. *Implant Dentistry, 13*(1), 11-19.

Stiell, I.G., et al. (2003). The Canadian C-spine rule versus the NEXUS low-risk criteria in patients with trauma. *New England Journal of Medicine, 349*(26), 2510-2518.

Todd, S.R. (2004). Critical concepts in abdominal injury. *Critical Care Clinics, 20*(1), 119-134.

Yealy, D.M., & Auble, T.E. Choosing between clinical prediction rules. *New England Journal of Medicine, 349*(26), 2553-2555.

Chapter 16

Sepsis and Septic Shock

Ruth M. Kleinpell

1. What is sepsis?

Sepsis is a complex clinical condition that results from increased inflammation, altered coagulation, and impaired fibrinolysis resulting from an infectious process. Mediator release induces endothelial damage, hypotension, and increased capillary permeability that result in impaired tissue perfusion and impaired cellular metabolism.

2. What are the risk factors for sepsis?

- Extremes of age: younger than 1 and older than 65 years of age
- Surgical and invasive procedures
- Endotracheal intubation and mechanical ventilation
- Presence of invasive catheters: Foley catheter, intravenous (IV) lines, surgical drains
- Malnutrition
- Broad-spectrum antibiotics
- Chronic illness
  - Diabetes mellitus
  - Chronic renal failure
  - Hepatitis
- Immunodeficiency disorders
- Compromised immune status
  - Acquired immunodeficiency syndrome
  - Use of cytotoxic and immunosuppressant agents
  - Alcoholism
  - Malignant neoplasms
  - Transplantation procedures
- Increase in the number of drug-resistant microorganisms

3. What is systemic inflammatory response syndrome (SIRS)?

SIRS is the systemic inflammatory response to a variety of severe clinical insults; the response is manifested by two or more of the following conditions:
- Temperature greater than 38° C (100.4° F) or less than 36° C (96.8° F)
- Heart rate greater than 90 beats/min

- Respiratory rate greater than 20 breaths/min or $Paco_2$ less than 32 mm Hg (<4.3 kPa)
- White blood cell (WBC) count greater than 12,000 cells/mm^3, less than 4000 cells/mm^3, or more than 10% immature (band) forms

4. How are sepsis, severe sepsis, and septic shock differentiated?

Sepsis is the systemic response to infection. Severe sepsis is sepsis involving organ system dysfunction, hypoperfusion, or hypotension. Septic shock is sepsis with hypotension, despite adequate fluid resuscitation, along with the presence of perfusion abnormalities that may include, but are not limited to, lactic acidosis, oliguria, or an acute alteration in mental status.

5. What hemodynamic changes are seen in sepsis?

Sepsis is characterized by a hyperdynamic state with increased central venous pressure and cardiac output. A decreased systemic vascular resistance is a hallmark of sepsis.

6. Identify the factors implicated in the development of multiple organ dysfunction syndrome (MODS) in severe sepsis.

- Tissue or organ hypoperfusion
- Ischemia
- Diffuse endothelial cellular injury
- Mediator release (e.g., tumor necrosis alpha, interleukin-1, platelet-activating factor, tissue factor, nitric oxide)
- Bacterial translocation
- Microthrombi
- Endothelial cell injury
- Alterations in vasomotor tone

7. What are the manifestations of organ system dysfunction in sepsis?

- *Respiratory dysfunction:* Alteration in oxygenation status, reflected by a decrease in the Pao_2/Fio_2 ratio or the need for supplemental oxygen ($Fio_2 \geq 0.40$); elevations in the level of positive end-expiratory pressure (≥ 5 to 10 mm H_2O);
  or the need for ventilatory assistance for 72 hours or more.
- *Cardiovascular dysfunction:* Hypotension, dysrhythmias, the need for inotropic or vasopressor support, and elevated filling pressures (e.g., central venous pressure, pulmonary capillary wedge pressure (PCWP).
- *Renal dysfunction:* Oliguria; serum creatinine levels greater than or equal to 2 mg/dL; need for dialysis or other replacement therapies to maintain fluid, acid-base, and electrolyte homeostasis.
- *Hematologic dysfunction:* Thrombocytopenia, leukocytosis or leukopenia, and biomarkers of coagulopathy, including abnormalities in the prothrombin time,

activated partial thromboplastin time, fibrin split products, D-dimer, or other evidence of disseminated intravascular coagulation.

- *Hepatic dysfunction:* Jaundice, hyperbilirubinemia, or elevated serum levels of hepatic enzymes, and less frequently as hypoalbuminemia or a prolonged prothrombin time. Liver failure may be defined by parameter gradations, including a serum bilirubin greater than 2 mg/dL for 48 hours with elevation of glutamate dehydrogenase to twice the normal level.
- *Gastrointestinal (GI) dysfunction:* GI bleeding, intolerance of enteral nutritional support, and intestinal ischemia or infarction, as well as less common manifestations, such as acalculous cholecystitis, pancreatitis, bowel perforation, ileus, and necrotizing enterocolitis.
- *Neurological dysfunction:* Confusion, agitation, and alterations in levels of consciousness.

8. What are treatment goals in sepsis?

- Appropriate antibiotic therapy has been found to reduce septic mortality by 10% to 15%. Empirical therapy with combination broad-spectrum (with or without Gram coverage) antibiotics should be initiated.
- Supportive treatment is with oxygenation and ventilation.
- Circulatory support is with fluid, vasopressor, and inotropic administration. The goal of fluid resuscitation is restoration of tissue perfusion and normalization of oxidative metabolism. Fluid infusion should be titrated to clinical endpoints, such as heart rate, blood pressure, and urine output.
- Vasopressive agents are indicated if maximum volume infusion (up to a PCWP of 15 to 18 mm Hg) does not normalize blood pressure and organ perfusion, as judged by a mean arterial pressure (MAP) greater than 60 mm Hg, adequate urine output, and normal organ function studies.
- Identification and eradication of infection source
- Culture surveillance
- Nutrition
- Stress ulcer prophylaxis
- Intensive insulin therapy
- Renal replacement therapy

9. What is the role of vasopressor in the treatment of septic shock?

The therapeutic goal of resuscitation is to maintain adequate organ perfusion, not pressure or total blood flow. Increasing perfusion pressure by a balanced increase in circulating blood volume and vasopressor therapy is the primary mechanism for increasing organ blood flow.

10. Identify some controversial therapies in the treatment of sepsis.

- Use of *dopamine* as a renal perfusion strategy. Several recent reviews including a meta-analysis of 58 studies and 19 randomized trials demonstrated no benefit of dopamine on reversing or preventing renal dysfunction, onset of acute renal failure, or need for dialysis (Kellum & Decker, 2001).

- Use of *norepinephrine* as a first-line agent. Recent data suggest that norepinephrine may be more advantageous than high-dose dopamine or epinephrine as a vasopressive agent in septic shock, improving arterial blood pressure, urine flow, and oxygen delivery (Martin et al., 2000).
- Use of *vasopressin.* Vasopressin has recently been used for refractory vasodilatory shock, although its use in shock is currently not an approved indication and the dosing guidelines are not firmly established (low doses of 0.1 to 1.0 units/min IV continuous are advocated).

11. **What are the most common sites of infection?**
    - Lung
    - Abdomen
    - Urinary tract

12. **Describe the indications for use of drotrecogin alpha (activated) therapy (Xigris) in severe sepsis.**

    Xigris is indicated for the treatment of severe sepsis with a high risk of mortality (e.g., as determined by scores on the Acute Physiology and Chronic Health Evaluation [APACHE] II). Indications for use include known or suspected infection, with at least three indications of SIRS and evidence of at least one organ system dysfunction. Xigris therapy has been shown to reduce mortality in patients with severe sepsis and organ failure within 48 hours of diagnosis.

13. **What are contraindications for use of Xigris therapy?**

    Contraindications for use of Xigris therapy include active bleeding or high risk for bleeding, due to the known profibrinolytic effects of Xigris therapy.

    Specific contraindications include the following:
    - Active internal bleeding (within 3 months)
    - Hemorrhagic stroke (within 2 months)
    - Severe head trauma
    - Intracranial or intraspinal surgery
    - Trauma with risk of life-threatening bleeding
    - Presence of epidural catheter
    - Intracranial neoplasm or mass lesion or evidence of cerebral herniation

14. **What is the role of steroids in severe sepsis?**

    Controversy regarding the use of steroid therapy in severe sepsis continues to exist. However, results from recent studies have shown beneficial effects of steroid use in patients with sepsis who have adrenal insufficiency (Yildiz et al., 2002; Annane et al., 2002).

15. What are sepsis prevention measures?

- Enforced infection control measures
- Handwashing
- Measures to prevent nosocomial infections
  - Oral care
  - Proper positioning (semirecumbent position during mechanical ventilation)
  - Turning and skin care
  - Invasive catheter care
  - Wound care
- Identifying patients at risk for sepsis
- Prioritizing cultures/pan cultures for febrile episodes
- Astute clinical assessment

Key Points

- Sepsis is the leading cause of death in intensive care patients.
- Cellulitis may progress to sepsis in the immunocompromised or older adult patient.
- Xigris is a new treatment for patients with severe sepsis.

Internet Resources

Sepsis.com:
www.sepsis.com

Society of Critical Care Medicine: Sepsis Guide:
www.sccm.org/press_room/sepsis_guide.asp

International Sepsis Forum:
www.sepsisforum.org

Bibliography

Annane, D., et al. (2002). Effect of treatment with low doses of hydrocortisone and fludrocortisone on mortality in patients with sepsis shock. *Journal of the American Medical Association, 268*, 862-871.

Balk, R.A., & Goyette, R.E. (2003). The multiple organ dysfunction syndrome in patients with severe sepsis: more than just inflammation. In R.A. Balk (Ed.). *Diagnosis and management of the patient with severe sepsis*. London: Royal Society of Medicine.

Balk, R.A. (2000). Pathogenesis and management of multiple organ dysfunction or failure in severe sepsis and septic shock. *Critical Care Clinics, 16*, 337-352.

Bernard, G.R., et al. (2001). Efficacy and safety of recombinant human activated protein C for severe sepsis. *New England Journal of Medicine, 344,* 699-709.

Berry, B.E. (2002). Assessing tissue oxygenation. *Critical Care Nursing, 22,* 22-42.

Ely, W., Kleinpell, R., & Goyette, R. (2003). Advances in the understanding and clinical manifestations and therapy of severe sepsis: An update for critical care nurses. *American Journal of Critical Care, 12,* 120-133.

Goodman, S., & Spring, C.L. (2002). The international sepsis forum's controversies in sepsis: Corticosteroids should be used to treat septic shock. *Critical Care, 6,* 381-383.

Harrison's Online. Shock. Accessed January 5, 2003, from http://www.harrisonsonline.com.

Jindal, N., Hollenberg, S.M., & Dellinger, R.P. (2000). Pharmacologic issues in the management of septic shock. *Critical Care Clinics, 16,* 233-249.

Kellum, J.A., & Decker, J.M. (2001). Use of dopamine in acute renal failure: A meta-analysis. *Critical Care Medicine, 29,* 1526-1531.

Kleinpell, R. (2003a). Advances in the management of the patient with severe sepsis: The role of drotrecogin alpha (activated). *Critical Care Nurse, 23,* 16-29.

Kleinpell, R. (2003b). The role of the critical care nurse in the assessment and management of the patient with severe sepsis. *Critical Care Nurse Quarterly, 15,* 27-34.

Kruse, J.A., Fink, M.P., & Carlson, R.W. (2003). *Saunders manual of critical care.* Philadelphia: W.B. Saunders.

Martin, C., et al. (2000). Effect of norepinephrine on the outcome of septic shock. *Critical Care Medicine, 28,* 2758-2765.

Rivers, E., et al. (2001). Early goal-directed therapy in the treatment of severe sepsis and septic shock. *New England Journal of Medicine, 345,* 1368-1377.

Schiffl, H., Lang, S.M., & Fischer, R. (2002). Daily hemodialysis and outcome of acute renal failure. *New England Journal of Medicine, 346,* 305-310.

Task Force of the American College of Critical Care Medicine. (1999). Practice parameters for hemodynamic support of sepsis in adult patients in sepsis. *Critical Care Medicine, 27,* 639-660.

van den Berghe, G., et al. (2001). Intensive insulin therapy in critically ill patients. *New England Journal of Medicine, 345,* 1359-1367.

Vervloet, M.G., Thijs, L.G., & Hack, C.E. (1998). Derangements of coagulation and fibrinolysis in critically ill patients with sepsis and septic shock. *Seminars in Thrombosis and Hemostasis, 24,* 33-44.

Wheeler, A.P., & Bernard, G.R. (1999). Treating patients with severe sepsis. *New England Journal of Medicine, 340,* 207-214.

Yildiz, O., et al. (2002). Physiological-dose steroid therapy in sepsis. *Critical Care, 6,* 251-259.

Xigris [package insert]. (2001). Indianapolis, IN: Eli Lilly.

Chapter 17

Advanced Cardiac Support Devices

Mary Lou O'Hara

1. What are the components of a good ventricular assist device (VAD) program?

The design of a VAD program depends on the institution's target population. VAD users range from hospitals with no cardiac surgery program to active cardiac transplantation centers. A quality program supporting a busy transplantation and cardiac surgical center requires an infrastructure that includes a variety of clinical disciplines. A recent analysis by Medicare regarding the support of a destination population provides a list of key individuals necessary for the support of this high acuity population. Central to any program is an advanced practice clinician who oversees the structure, consults with a variety of disciplines in the care of these patients, coordinates discharge planning and outpatient support, and provides teaching to both patient and staff.

2. What are the criteria for placement of a VAD?

Currently the main criteria for placing a patient on a cardiac assist device are as follows:
- Class IV heart failure unresponsive to maximal medical therapy
- Support for a reversible cardiac event that results in shock such as nonseparation from cardiopulmonary bypass (CPB) or cardiogenic shock associated with an acute myocardial infarction (AMI)
- Permanent support for patients not considered transplant candidates

3. What are the physiological principles of ventricular assistance?

- Support for stunned myocardium
- Reduction of wall tension
- Improvement in myocardial oxygen consumption
- Restoration of adenosine triphosphate (ATP) stores
- Support circulation
- Reverse acidosis
- Restore end-organ function
- Reduce need for inotropes

4. Are there contraindications to implanting a VAD?

In the bridge to transplant population, the following *may* be considered contraindications but are evaluated on a case-by-case basis. However, in the patient in whom the mechanical device is the final treatment, age and comorbidities that would make a patient ineligible for transplant are *not* definite contraindications:

- Recent or irreversible neurological injury
- Active systemic infection
- Evidence of irreversible end-organ function
- Aortic insufficiency greater than +2
- Lack of social support
- Active addiction history
- Active malignancy
- Age older than 70 years
- Morbid obesity (body mass index >30%)

5. How are these pumps powered and how do they provide flow?

Pumps either mimic physiological function by providing a dynamic pulsatile flow or a continuous flow of blood in a nonpulsatile stream.

Pulsatile pumps propel blood forward, either pushed by a bolus of compressed air (e.g., Abiomed BVS 5000 or Thoratec PVAD) or pushed by an electrically powered assembly such as a flexing diaphragm or pusher plate (e.g., Thoratec HeartMate or World Heart Novacor).

Nonpulsatile flow is provided by tubing compressed by a rotating roller (typically used in a cardiopulmonary bypass circuit); centrifugal force provided by a rapidly rotating blade or cone (e.g., Biomedicus or Sarns); or a rotating impeller similar to a boat propeller (e.g., Jarvik 2000 or Micromed DeBakey).

6. What VADs are currently in use?

Current Food and Drug Administration (FDA)-approved devices are all pulsatile and include the following:

ABIOMED BVS 5000 (see figure on p. 201)
The Abiomed is a system consisting of inflow and outflow cannulas, connecting tubing, and an external two-chambered blood pump connected to a pneumatic console. Unidirectional flow is provided by two incorporated valves at the exit from each chamber. The BVS 5000 provides up to 6.5 L of pulsatile blood flow and requires anticoagulation. The pump can provide either single or biventricular support. It is indicated for short-term use as a bridge to recovery or bridge to another longer term device.

THORATEC PARACORPOREAL (see figure on p. 202)
The Thoratec PVAD is a pulsatile, pneumatically driven pump providing up to 7 L of flow in either a univentricular or biventricular configuration. The Thoratec is approved as both a bridge to recovery and a bridge to transplant. Inflow and outflow cannulas exit the chest and are attached to a compressible blood sac contained in solid polycarbonate housing. Unidirectional flow is provided by two Bjork-Shiley tilting disc valves that require anticoagulation. The pump is

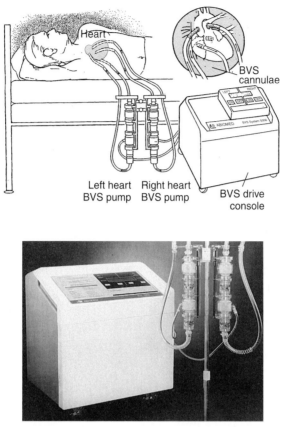

Abiomed BVS 5000. *(Reprinted with permission of Abiomed, Danvers, MA).*

powered by either a large dual-drive pneumatic console or a smaller portable driver called the TLC-II. Patient discharge on the TLC-II has recently been approved by the FDA.

THORATEC HEARTMATE (see figure on p. 202)
The HeartMate is a left ventricular assist device (LVAD) approved as a bridge to transplant and recently as permanent support (destination). Two models (pneumatic and electric) are available; both allow complete patient mobility. An inflow cannula containing a porcine valve is attached to the left ventricular (LV) apex and another valve conduit is attached to a Dacron graft anastomosed to the ascending aorta. Both conduits traverse the diaphragm and are attached to a two-chambered titanium pump. The blood contacting chamber has a roughened internal surface of titanium and textured polyurethane that encourages the layering of a pseudoendothelial lining. This surface, in combination with the biological valves, avoids the use of anticoagulation. The flexing diaphragm is propelled by either a pusher plate (pneumatic design) or a rotating cam (electric). The pump is placed either intra-abdominally or in a surgically

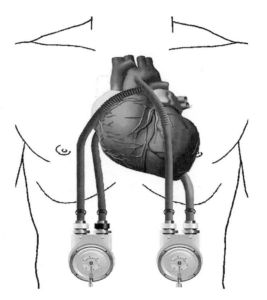

Thoratec Paracorporeal shown in BiVAD configuration. *(Reprinted with permission of Thoratec, Pleasanton, CA.)*

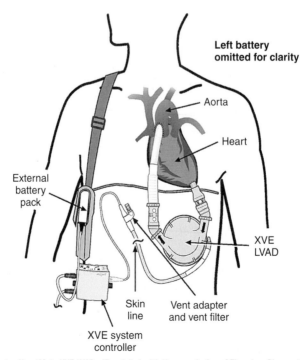

Thoratec HeartMate XVE LVAD. *(Reprinted with the permission of Thoratec, Pleasanton, CA.)*

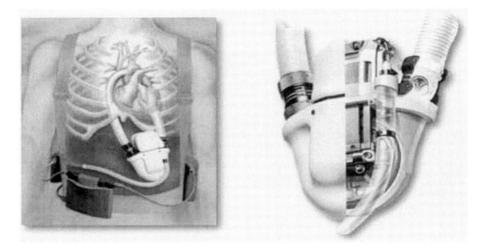

World Heart Novacor LVAS. *Left,* Patient configuration. *Right,* Novacor LVAS. *(Reprinted with permission of World Heart, Oakland, CA.)*

fashioned preperitoneal pocket and power is provided via an external driveline. The pump can provide up to 10 L of flow.

WORLD HEART NOVACOR (see figure above)
The Novacor pump is an electrically powered LVAD approved as a bridge to transplant and is currently in an FDA trial to determine its potential for permanent support. Its cannula conduits contain biological valves attached to a blood sac housed within a solid external shell. Two symmetrically aligned plates compress the blood sac and provide a maximum stroke volume of 70 mL and up to 10 L of flow. Anticoagulation is required.

7. How should one choose a VAD for any given patient?

Surgical decisions in choosing a VAD include the following:
- Patient presentation and history
- Assumed length of support
- Size of patient
- Anatomical variants
- Consideration for home support

Right and left ventricular function is evaluated to determine the need for either univentricular (RVAD or LVAD) or biventricular (BiVAD) support. Indications for BiVAD support may include the following:
- Intractable dysrhythmias
- RV/septal infarct
- Elevated pulmonary vascular resistance (PVR)
- Right-sided heart failure (RHF)
- Prolonged shock
- "Sicker patients"

8. **What are the common modes of VAD operation?**

Pulsatile VADs function in either an automatic fill to empty mode or in a fixed mode. Both provide flow asynchronous to native electrical activity.

In an *automatic mode,* a sensor is triggered when the blood contacting chamber is filled to a preprogrammed percent of its fill capacity. As preload increases, the VAD speeds up its rate until it reaches its upper rate limit. As preload declines, the VAD slows until it reaches its base rate. Changes in afterload can also affect the rate response of a VAD due to the effect on VAD emptying.

In *fixed mode,* the clinician determines a rate that will provide the flow (in liters per minute) required for the clinical situation. The fixed rate mode is used in the following situations:
- In the operating room when first powering on, thus providing a controlled transition off CPB.
- In the patient who is recovering myocardial function (e.g., postcardiotomy). By setting a fixed rate, thus a controlled flow, the patient's ventricle is gradually reintroduced to loading conditions to determine readiness for explantation. The clinician then monitors response via an echocardiogram (ECHO) as well as hemodynamic data analysis.
- In the setting of a regurgitant valve (either the pump or native valves), the pump rate is artificially high due to the recirculation of blood. Depending on the ratio of forward to regurgitant flow, this can cause significant hemodynamic compromise if native ventricular function is severely depressed. This situation could also cause significant wear on the pump mechanics. By setting a fixed rate appropriate to provide adequate forward flow and hemodynamic support, less damage to the pump is achieved until a definitive solution (transplant, explant, or pump exchange) to the problem is determined.

9. **Are there backup systems in case of power failure?**

All FDA-approved pumps have backup systems, either in the form of emergency power sources or manual hand pumps. Refer to the manufacturer's directions for use (DFU).

10. **What is involved in the preoperative evaluation of a patient for VAD implant?**

Depending on whether the implant is emergent or elective, the preoperative workup may include the following:
- History and physical and precipitating events leading to current status
- ECHO

11. **What is involved in the preoperative preparation of a patient for VAD implant?**

- Skin preparation with antiseptic scrub
- Nutritional analysis to include prealbumin and transferrin
- Evaluation of renal and liver function

- Oral/dental examination and care
- Psychosocial evaluation
- Nasal Bactroban (to reduce nosocomial methicillin-resistant *Streptococcus aureus* infection)
- Determination of previous chest surgery or radiation to prepare for adequate blood products and anticipate potential for chest entry complication
- Prophylactic antibiotics per institutional protocol, usually avoiding aminoglycosides because of potential for renal impairment
- Cytomegalovirus (CMV) status to determine the need for CMV-free blood products in pretransplant patients
- Leukocyte-depleted blood products in pretransplant patients
- History of previous exposure to aprotinin (used to decrease bleeding complications) because reexposure can create an anaphylactic reaction
- Evaluation of dysrhythmia and current therapy
- Determination of presence of an automated internal cardiac defibrillator (AICD) or pacemaker

12. Why is a preoperative ECHO important?

To prepare the patient for the appropriate surgical approach, an ECHO provides critical information for the surgeon:
- Identifies a right-to-left shunt patent foramen ovale (PFO) which, if unrecognized, can cause profound hypoxemia
- Identifies valvular problems
- Identifies a left ventricular or left atrial thrombus
- Identifies an ascending aorta atheroma; although difficult to see on ECHO, the presence of atheroma may determine alternate positioning of an LVAD outflow cannula
- Determines right ventricular function
- Determines conduit position

13. How is a VAD implanted?

Paracorporeal VADs have cannulas that exit the skin subcostally and are externally connected to the blood pump.

Intracorporeal (HeartMate and Novacor) pumps are implanted below the diaphragm, either intra-abdominally or in a surgically fashioned preperitoneal pocket, depending on the surgeon's preference and experience.

14. Describe the considerations related to choice of cannula placement.

Decisions regarding cannulation, atrial or ventricular (see figures on p. 206), depend on the device used, the type of cannula available, and the clinical setting. Considerations related to cannula choice include the following:
Ventricular
- Lower risk of thromboembolism
- Higher VAD flows
- Better option for myocardial recovery due to LV decompression

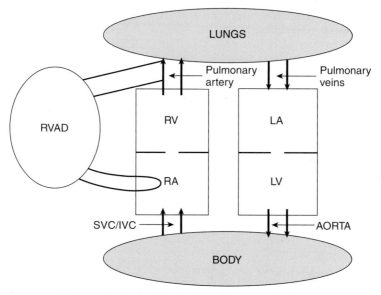

RVAD schematic showing inflow from RA out to pump and outflow to PA.

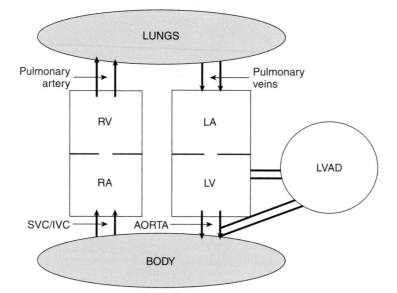

LVAD schematic showing inflow from LV and out to pump and outflow to aorta.

Atrial
- Easy to insert/remove
- Minimal dissection
- No CPB required
- Avoids infarct/thrombus/aneurysm
- May be a better option for explant

15. What are the main perioperative issues related to VAD insertion?
- Availability of echocardiography
- Preoperative clinical status
- Preperitoneal or intra-abdominal placement
- Protection of the right ventricle

16. What parameters are measured postoperatively?
- Right-sided heart function
- Pulmonary vascular resistance
- Systemic vascular resistance
- Cardiac rhythm
- Peripheral perfusion
- LVAD output in relation to thermodilution cardiac output
- Perioperative hemodynamics and findings
- Coagulation panel and give blood product–specific therapy as indicated

17. What are the most significant factors in postoperative management?
- Following monitoring trends
- Managing comorbidities
- Managing bleeding

18. What complications should be anticipated?
Along with those complications related to cardiac surgery and CPB, such as bleeding and tamponade, the complications of greatest concern in the VAD-supported patient include the following:
- RV dysfunction (in patients with LVAD only)
- Infection
- Decreased LVAD output
- Mechanical malfunction

19. What is the differential diagnosis when evaluating low VAD output?
- Physiological contributors to decreased LVAD output
  - Hypovolemia
  - Bleeding
  - Tamponade
  - RV failure

- Pulmonary hypertension
- Dysrhythmia
- Mechanical contributors to decreased LVAD output
  - Inflow obstruction
  - Outflow obstruction
  - Interference with power supply
  - Leaks in system (pneumatic systems)

20. What interventions are used to optimize RV dysfunction?

- Reduce RV afterload.
  - Avoidance of hypoxia and acidosis
  - Use of inodilators (milrinone, dobutamine)
  - Use of inhaled afterload agents such as nitric oxide or prostacyclin
  - Control of bleeding
  - Careful volume loading
  - Use of a fixed rate setting to minimize RV overload and preserve ventricular septal geometry
- Treat ischemia.
- Treat dysrhythmias.
- Monitor right atrial pressure (RAP) and pulmonary artery pressure (PAP).
- Reevaluate with ECHO as indicated.

21. How is cardiac tamponade recognized and treated?

Evaluation of tamponade can be challenging in the post-VAD patient and can occur late in the postoperative course, particularly in patients requiring anticoagulation. Compression of cardiac structures or graft conduits can result from coagulopathic bleeding, poorly controlled anticoagulation, or disruption of suture lines. Late bleeding can also occur as a result of an infectious process disrupting graft or suture integrity. As with all cardiac surgical patients, ongoing vigilance is key. Decreasing VAD flows, dropping hemoglobin, and rising RAP, as well as indications of systemic hypoperfusion are all possible reflections of tamponade physiology. Diagnosis can be aided by use of an ECHO. Maintaining an active type-and-screen for immediate availability of blood products is recommended. Reoperation may be indicated if hemodynamic compromise is evident.

22. What infection prophylaxis should be considered?

The threat of infection is always present when there is a large biological interface as well as when cannulas traverse the skin:

- Antibiotics for 48 to 72 hours postoperatively
- Removal of central lines and Foley catheter early in the postoperative period
- Meticulous oral care
- Oral nystatin if the patient is receiving antibiotics
- Early culture for
  - Any temperature greater than 100.6° F

- Any white blood cell count greater than 11,000 cells/mm^3 and rising
- Any characteristic change in cannula site indicative of infectious process
- Meticulous cannula site care, including
  - Strict aseptic technique
  - Dressing care at intervals appropriate to cannula type and site
  - Increased frequency of dressing change to avoid wet dressing
  - Immobilization, which is key to good tissue in-growth

23. How are dysrhythmias treated?

The approach to dysrhythmia treatment is based on the significance of the hemodynamic effect of the dysrhythmia. Remarkably, many LVAD patients tolerate ventricular tachycardia as long as forward blood flow is maintained. This may allow the clinician time to load with an antidysrhythmic agent or electively prepare for cardioversion. In BiVAD patients, organized rhythm is less important unless ventricular recovery is anticipated.

24. Can the electronics of the VAD be harmed if an AICD is triggered?

The energy of an AICD is not high enough to damage the electrical circuitry of the current FDA-approved VADs.

Perioperatively, the AICD is off. If dealing with a patient on BiVAD support, it is often policy to leave the AICD off. If the patient is on an LVAD, it is important to maintain electrical stability. Therefore, the AICD function is restored post-operatively. Reinterrogation by electrophysiology study is indicated to evaluate any changes required as a result of perioperative events.

25. What is the process for cardioversion?

For the Abiomed and Thoratec paracorporeal (PVAD), there is no danger of interfering with the electronics of the VAD system and cardioversion/defibrillation can be done safely. In a patient with a Thoratec HeartMate, however, the electronic circuitry of the external system controller could be damaged. Power and the external controller are removed, and the patient's heart is hand-pumped during the procedure.

26. Is anticoagulation necessary with all VADs?

Most FDA-approved VADs (except the HeartMate) require anticoagulation. Typically, a heparin drip is initiated once coagulation parameters are normalized after CPB, usually within 12 hours postoperatively and once chest tube output has diminished to less than 50 mL/hr. Depending on the institution and device, activating clotting time (ACT) or partial thromboplastin time (PTT) is used to track heparin activity. More recently, thromboelastograms, which measure rate and strength of clot formation, are becoming a helpful adjunct to heparin monitoring. Target goals are set according to the postoperative period and which ventricular chambers are supported. In some institutions, the goal range for

BiVAD-supported patients is higher than for single ventricular support. Once the platelet count has normalized, antiplatelet therapy is initiated. Transition to warfarin (Coumadin) may be considered once the patient's nutritional status has been optimized.

27. How are patients managed who develop heparin-induced thrombocytopenia (HIT)?

Once HIT is confirmed (facilitated by a thorough hematologic workup), heparin analogues, such as lepirudin or argatroban, may be used. Monitoring is difficult because PTT and ACT are not specific reflections of these drugs' activities. Doses must be carefully adjusted in the setting of either renal or liver dysfunction.

28. If treating a patient whose therapeutic goal is recovery and explant, what are the indications of improved native ventricular function?

Typically, evidence of native recovery is confirmed by ECHO. Unlike the asynchronous pulse wave generated by the VAD, phasic evidence of native ventricular ejection can be visible on an arterial line trace in synchrony with the native rhythm (see figure below). Depending upon how vigorously native ejection contributes to cardiac output, VAD flows may be low despite a stable hemodynamic profile.

29. How is recovery optimized?

Once recovery potential is evident, adjunctive pharmacological therapy may be helpful. Angiotensin-converting enzyme inhibitors or angiotensin receptor blocking therapy and other mainstays of heart failure management may be considered if the etiology of the ventricular function warrants. A period of gradual ventricular loading may be attempted while monitoring hemodynamics and oxygenation. Increases in anticoagulation may be required as VAD flow is strategically reduced. Once the decision to explant has been reached, additional inotropic and inodilator therapy may be required to facilitate the transition from VAD support to independent ventricular function.

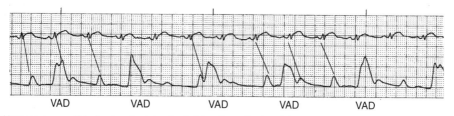

VAD   VAD   VAD   VAD   VAD

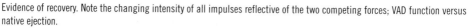

Evidence of recovery. Note the changing intensity of all impulses reflective of the two competing forces; VAD function versus native ejection.

30. **What resources are there to assist in the management of VAD-supported patients?**

In centers without a formal VAD program, the various manufacturers have regional clinical specialists who are expert in the management and trouble-shooting of VADs. Each institution should be provided with a 24-hour access number in case of emergency. There are also resources on the Internet. It is also helpful to contact other VAD centers and speak with an experienced clinician.

31. **How is discharge potential for a VAD-supported patient determined?**

Home discharge is remarkably feasible and helpful in patients who have the ability to cope with the mechanical device and whose wait for transplant may be long. Since the FDA has approved the HeartMate for permanent support, discharge planning has become a regular aspect of the VAD program.

Once the patient is medically stable and cognitive function allows for intensification of the educational process, programmed instruction is introduced to the patient and family. In patients who are electively scheduled for an implant, education can occur preoperatively.

A thorough evaluation of the home environment is completed and encompasses architectural features of the home, including any electrical or general safety concerns. Communication is initiated with the home community including the primary care provider, EMS, and local hospital. Before the patient is discharged, a series of day passes is helpful to evaluate the effectiveness of the training and readiness of the patient for independent living. Use of beepers and cell phones are highly recommended so emergency communication is facilitated.

32. **What travel considerations are necessary for a patient with a VAD?**

Once the patient has been home and stable, the team can entertain the appropriate timing for travel beyond the community. A patient's transplant status may determine how far the patient can travel. If more extensive travel is planned, coordination with the destination community is important. The risks of traveling, particularly outside the United States, must be discussed. If possible, communication with a VAD center in the destination region provides a cushion of safety. If traveling by air, elaborate planning and collaboration with airlines and airport security is crucial.

33. **What adverse effects can be expected during long-term VAD support?**

Wear and tear of mechanical moving parts is inevitable and, in the destination population, is a predictable future event. Postoperative follow-up should always consider the possibility of a disruption in the function of the device. Examination of external components as well as a memory of the acoustic signature is helpful in anticipating a disruption in the mechanics. Inflow and outflow valves can become regurgitant, causing a high rate and flow, potentially causing more wear on internal parts.

Infection remains a constant risk as long as percutaneous lines are required for energy transfer. And, because the home environment and patient activities cannot be controlled by the nurse, patient injury from imprudent activity is always a concern.

34. What types of VADs are expected to be seen in the future?

Nearly 50 devices are in the research and development stage internationally. Scientists and engineers are constantly striving to develop smaller devices that will have an expanded functional life. A number of devices have eliminated percutaneous drivelines, and newer axial and centrifugal devices are significantly smaller. Clinicians need to be ready for the impact these new nonpulsatile devices will have on aspects of physical assessment and care. The era of the bionic man and woman is here.

Key Points

- VADs are systems that either support or take over failing ventricular function.
- The majority of current FDA-approved devices are pulsatile, mimicking physiological function.
- Choice of a VAD depends on patient history and presentation, patient size, proposed length of support, and the need for either single or biventricular support.
- VAD flow is provided at either a predetermined fixed rate or in an automatic mode that responds to changes in preload.
- Echocardiography provides essential information at implant and can assist the clinician in postoperative monitoring of complications.
- Anticoagulation is required for most FDA-approved VADs; an exception is the Thoratec HeartMate.
- The most common complications of VADs are infection and bleeding.
- Preparation for discharge of a VAD-supported patient requires a comprehensive program that includes extensive patient teaching as well as evaluation of the home environment and support network.
- Successful VAD programs are collaborative, multidisciplinary teams that include physicians, advance practice nurses, primary nurses, social workers, physical therapists, nutritionists, and engineers.

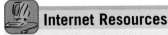

Internet Resources

Thoratec Corporation:
www.thoratec.com

Abiomed, Inc.:
www.abiomed.com

World Heart Corporation:
www.worldheart.com

Center for Medicare and Medicaid Services:
www.cms.hhs.gov

Bibliography

Christensen, D.M. (2000).The ventricular assist device: An overview. *Nursing Clinics of North America, 35*(4), 945-959.

Dew, M.A., et al. (2001). Quality of life outcomes after heart transplantation in individuals bridged to transplant with ventricular assist devices. *Journal of Heart and Lung Transplantation, 20,* 1199-1212.

Entwistle, J.W., 3rd. (2004). Short- and long-term mechanical ventricular assistance towards myocardial recovery. *Surgical Clinics of North America, 84*(1), 201-221.

Etoch, S.W., et al. (2003). Inhaled milrinone and prostacyclin for ventricular assist device recipients: Effectiveness and cost. *Journal of Heart and Lung Transplantation Supplement, 22*(2), 202-209.

Farrar, D.J. (2000). The Thoratec ventricular assist device: A paracorporeal pump for treating acute and chronic heart failure. *Seminars in Thoracic and Cardiovascular Surgery, 12,* 243-250.

Jaski, B.E., et al. (2001). Cardiac transplant outcome of patients supported on left ventricular assist device vs. intravenous inotropic therapy. *Journal of Heart and Lung Transplantation, 20,* 449-456.

Moskowitz, A.J., et al. (2001). The cost of long-term LVAD implantation. *Annals of Thoracic Surgery, 7,*:S195-S198.

Samuels, L. (2004). Biventricular mechanical replacement. *Surgical Clinics of North America, 84*(1), 309-321.

Ungerleider, R.M., et al. (2004). Routine mechanical ventricular assist following the Norwood procedure— Improved neurological outcome and excellent hospital survival. *Annals of Thoracic Surgery, 77*(1), 18-22.

Chapter 18

Classifications of Shock

Ruth M. Kleinpell

1. **Define shock.**

   Shock is a clinical condition that results in inadequate tissue perfusion and impaired cellular oxygenation. As the body's response to injury, trauma, or infection, shock results in systemic hypotension, acidosis, and impaired organ functioning.

2. **What are the clinical manifestations of shock?**

   - Hypotension
   - Tachycardia
   - Tachypnea
   - Pale, cool clammy skin
   - Oliguria
   - Decreased cardiac output

3. **Name the five types of shock.**

   - Hypovolemic
   - Cardiogenic
   - Anaphylactic
   - Neurogenic
   - Septic

   Anaphylactic, neurogenic, and septic shock are sometimes classified under the category of distributive shock.

4. **What are the body's compensatory mechanisms for shock?**

   Compensatory mechanisms for shock involve neuroendocrine responses, which are activated via atrial, arterial, and renal baroreceptor recognition of changes in vascular volume. These include the following:
   - Sympathetic nervous system release of the catecholamines epinephrine and norepinephrine, which promote increased contractility and heart rate.
   - Release of antidiuretic hormone and aldosterone to induce renal absorption of sodium and water to increase vascular volume.

- Renin-angiotensin–induced vasoconstriction.
- Increased adrenocorticotropic hormone (ACTH) secretion by the anterior pituitary, stimulating cortisol secretion by the adrenal cortex. Cortisol alters cellular metabolism, enhances lipolysis, and increases gluconeogenesis, increasing blood osmolarity and shifting fluid from the intracellular space to the intravascular space to increase circulating blood volume.

5. What are goals of treatment in shock?

The overall goals of treatment are aimed at increasing tissue perfusion and providing organ support. These include improving hemodynamics by increasing vascular volume, increasing blood pressure, and improving cardiac output and contractility. Specific measures include hemodynamic support with fluids, inotropic agents, and vasoconstrictive agents; oxygenation support with mechanical ventilation as needed; and other organ specific support including renal, gastrointestinal, hepatic, and hematological. Patients in shock should be treated in the intensive care unit with continuous electrocardiographic and arterial O_2 monitoring. Treatment should be titrated to clinical endpoints of blood pressure, heart rate, urine output, skin perfusion, mental status, and indices of tissue perfusion.

6. What are common causes of hypovolemic shock?

Common causes of hypovolemic shock include blood loss from trauma, gastrointestinal bleeding, burns, dehydration, massive gastrointestinal fluid losses from vomiting, diarrhea, nasogastric suctioning, and internal third spacing seen in ascites, bowel obstruction, and pancreatitis.

7. What are the clinical manifestations of hypovolemic shock?

Common signs of hypovolemic shock include tachycardia, hypotension, cold, clammy skin, and restlessness or agitation. Progressive signs include marked tachycardia, refractory hypotension, cardiac dysrhythmias, and signs of severely impaired tissue perfusion including acidosis and organ system dysfunction.

8. When are manifestations of hypovolemic shock evident?

Clinical manifestations of hypovolemic shock are seen when volume loss is at least 1500 mL or when volume loss is greater than 20% of circulating volume.

9. What are the stages of hypovolemic shock?

- *Initial stage:* 15% or 750 mL of volume loss. Compensatory mechanisms maintain the cardiac output, and the patient is asymptomatic.
- *Second or compensatory stage:* 15% to 30% (750 mL to 1500 mL) volume loss. Cardiac output falls and clinical signs of shock are evident: tachycardia, hypotension, decreased urine output, altered level of consciousness.

- *Third or progressive stage:* 30% to 40% (1500 mL to 2000 mL) volume loss. Compensatory mechanisms fail to maintain perfusion and severe impaired tissue perfusion results. It will result in severe hypotension, tachycardia, dysrhythmias, and metabolic acidosis.
- *Fourth or refractory stage:* Greater than 40% (>2000 mL) volume loss. It results in deterioration of compensatory mechanisms, organ failure, and cardiac arrest.

10. What are indicated aspects of management of hypovolemic shock?

Treatment of hypovolemic shock includes volume replacement and identification and treatment of the cause of volume loss. Controversy exists regarding the preferred replacement fluid: crystalloids or colloids. Initially, isotonic crystalloid solution, such as lactated Ringer's (LR) or normal saline solution is given. Colloids such as albumin and plasma substitutes (dextran, hetastarch) are also then used as volume expanders to replace lost intravascular volume.

Fluid resuscitation often follows a 3:1 rule: replace fluid losses with 3 mL of crystalloid or colloid for each 1 mL of volume loss. Packed red blood cell (PRBC) transfusions are indicated for a hematocrit (Hct) less than 28%. For each unit of PRBCs, expect an increase of 3% in Hct and 1 g/dL increase in hemoglobin (Hgb). When typed and cross-matched blood is unavailable, universal donor type O, Rh-negative blood is administered.

11. What are common causes of cardiogenic shock?

- Acute myocardial infarction
- Pulmonary edema
- Cardiomyopathies
- Dysrhythmias
- Pericardial tamponade
- Valvular regurgitation

12. What are the clinical manifestations of cardiogenic shock?

- Tachycardia
- Hypotension
- Pale, cool, clammy skin
- Oliguria
- Distended neck veins

13. What are hemodynamic indicators of cardiogenic shock?

The clinical definition of cardiogenic shock is a decreased cardiac output with evidence of tissue hypoxia in the presence of adequate intravascular volume. The hemodynamic criteria for cardiogenic shock include sustained hypotension with a systolic blood pressure less than 90 mm Hg for at least 30 minutes and a reduced cardiac index of less than 2.2 L/min per m^2 with a pulmonary capillary wedge pressure greater than 15 mm Hg.

14. What type of myocardial dysfunction is present in cardiogenic shock?

Cardiogenic shock is characterized by both systolic and diastolic myocardial dysfunction. Impaired left ventricular ejection leads to increased left end-diastolic pressure and pulmonary congestion, which can progress to diastolic dysfunction. In cardiogenic shock, cardiac output and stroke volume are decreased, causing decreased systemic perfusion, hypotension, and compensatory vasoconstriction and fluid retention. Progressive myocardial dysfunction results in inadequate tissue perfusion, cellular hypoxia, and ischemia.

15. What are treatment goals in cardiogenic shock?

* Increase cardiac output
* Enhance contractility
* Correct dysrhythmias
* Optimize the heart rate
* Increase myocardial oxygen delivery
* Decrease oxygen demands

These goals, however, can be clinically challenging to achieve, in that interventions to increase cardiac output and contractility tend to also increase myocardial oxygen demands.

16. Describe the treatment plans for cardiogenic shock.

Treatment components include supplemental oxygenation, hemodynamic support, diuretics for pulmonary congestion, and fluid resuscitation for hypotension only if pulmonary edema is present. Positive inotropic agents (beta-adrenergics) are given to increase contractility (dobutamine, dopamine). Vasodilators may be used to decrease left ventricular afterload (nitroglycerin; nitroprusside); however, vasodilator therapy can compromise blood pressure and dosages must be titrated cautiously.

Intra-aortic balloon pump (IABP) counterpulsation may be indicated to augment coronary artery perfusion pressure (inflation during diastole) and to decrease left ventricular afterload (deflation just before ventricular systole).

When hypotension remains refractory, catecholamines (norepinephrine) may be necessary to maintain organ perfusion. However, catecholamine infusions must be carefully titrated in patients with cardiogenic shock to maximize coronary perfusion pressure with the least possible increase in myocardial oxygen demand. Vasopressin has recently been used for refractory vasodilatory shock, although its use in cardiogenic shock is currently not an approved indication and the dosing guidelines are not firmly established (low doses of 0.1 to 1.0 units/min intravenously continuous are advocated).

Revascularization and reperfusion interventions may also be indicated for cardiogenic shock. The SHOCK trial demonstrated that early reperfusion strategies (angioplasty, coronary artery bypass surgery) within 6 hours of cardiogenic shock resulting from acute myocardial infarction improved survival rates (Hochman et al., 1999).

17. Describe anaphylactic shock.

Anaphylactic shock results from an allergic reaction, which causes systemic release of immunoglobulin E (antibody formed as part of immune response) that results in direct activation of mast cells and histamine release. Histamine, along with other mediators such as prostaglandins, kinins, and complement, cause vasodilation, increased vascular permeability, bronchoconstriction, and coronary vasoconstriction. The result is peripheral pooling of blood, tissue edema, airway constriction, and myocardial depression, which can progress and cause altered tissue perfusion and impaired cellular metabolism.

18. What are the clinical manifestations of anaphylactic shock?

The clinical manifestations of anaphylactic shock include generalized pruritus, urticaria (hives), angioedema (edema of lips/tongue), respiratory distress, syncope, and apprehension.

19. What are common allergens?

Common allergens that can induce anaphylactic shock include foods, food additives, drugs, hormones, serum products (gamma globulin), blood products, vaccines, venoms, dust, pollen, and latex.

20. What are routes of entry for allergens?

- Injection
- Ingestion
- Inhalation
- Skin absorption

21. When are manifestations of anaphylactic shock seen?

Anaphylactic shock is a life-threatening hypersensitivity reaction, which can develop rapidly (within seconds) or occur as a delayed response (12 or more hours after initial exposure). The severity of the reaction is directly related to the onset of symptoms, with early signs appearing with a severe reaction. Occasionally, biphasic reactions occur in which symptoms recur several hours after the initial reaction.

22. What are treatment goals for anaphylactic shock?

- ABCs of emergency care (airway, breathing, and circulation)
- Volume expansion
- Hypotension managed with intravenous crystalloids or colloid solutions to promote intravascular volume expansion
- Vasoconstrictor agents to reverse the effects of severe vasodilation and depressed myocardial function

23. What vasoconstrictors may be used in treatment of anaphylactic shock?

- *Epinephrine* is a first-line drug given to patients with anaphylaxis as it promotes bronchodilation and vasoconstriction and inhibits further mediator release. Epinephrine is given in a standard dose of 0.01 mL/kg of a 1:1000 solution, up to a maximum of 0.3 to 0.5 mL, given subcutaneously every 10 to 20 minutes until the patient is stabilized. In life-threatening reactions with severe shock, intravenous administration of epinephrine may be required. The dose for intravenous epinephrine is 0.1 to 0.5 mg of a 1:10,000 solution, which is repeated in 10-minute intervals (not to exceed 0.5 mg in 10 minutes).
- *Antihistamines* (such as diphenhydramine [Benadryl]) are useful as a second-line drug therapy to block the histamine response and stop the inflammatory reaction.
- *Aminophylline* and inhaled beta$_2$ agonists may be used to reverse bronchospasm.
- *Corticosteroids* (such as methylprednisolone [Solu-Medrol]) may be given to help stabilize capillary membranes and prevent delayed reaction.

24. What are preventive measures for patients at risk for anaphylactic shock?

- Avoid the allergen.
- Wear Medical Alert identification.
- Read food ingredients.
- Ask about food preparation when eating out.
- Be aware of subtle symptoms that may indicate a reaction.
- Seek prompt medical attention when symptoms occur.
- Carry and use self-administered epinephrine for emergency reactions.

25. What is neurogenic shock?

Neurogenic shock results from loss of sympathetic vasomotor tone, causing arteriolar and venous dilation, decreased afterload and preload with subsequent vasodilation and decreased cardiac output. Unopposed vagal tone can result in significant bradycardia.

26. What are causes of neurogenic shock?

Neurogenic shock is caused predominantly from acute spinal cord injury, specifically cervical and upper thoracic spinal cord injuries. Neurogenic shock can also result from regional anesthesia or autonomic blocking agents, although the occurrence is infrequent.

27. What are the clinical manifestations of neurogenic shock?

- Hypotension
- Light-headedness
- Weakness
- Bradycardia (or reflex tachycardia)
- Pale, cool, clammy skin with warm extremities above the level of injury
- Decreased level of consciousness

28. What are treatment goals for neurogenic shock?

- ABCs of emergency care.
- Fluid resuscitation for hypotension, but with caution because blood volume is sufficient and shock is related to altered blood distribution.
- Supine or Trendelenburg positioning to promote reestablishment of blood pressure and cerebral perfusion.
- Atropine to block dominant vagal effects causing bradycardia.
- Vasoconstrictive intravenous agents or positive inotropic agents to enhance cardiac output and perfusion pressure and improve renal hemodynamics. However, vasopressors should be used with caution because vasoconstriction may decrease spinal cord blood flow, which can ultimately influence the extent of secondary cord injury.
- Pacemaker for refractory bradydysrhythmias.
- Insertion of a Foley catheter if bladder function is lost.

Key Points

- Always look for reversible causes of shock.
- Distributive shock is associated with a low peripheral vascular resistance.
- The goal in treatment of shock is to normalize tissue oxygen delivery.

Internet Resources

EMedicine: Shock, Cardiogenic:
www.emedicine.com/EMERG/topic530.htm

Critical Care Medicine Tutorials: Treating Septic Shock:
www.ccmtutorials.com/infection/sepsisrx

Critical Care Medicine Tutorials: Shock Introduction:
www.ccmtutorials.com/cvs/Shock/page_01.htm

Bibliography

Albright, T.N., Zimmerman, M.A., & Selzman, C.H. (2002). Vasopressin in the cardiac surgery intensive care unit. *American Journal of Critical Care, 11,* 326-332.

American College of Surgeons, Committee on Trauma. (2000). *Advanced trauma life support student course manual.* Chicago: Author.

Balk, R.A. (2000). Pathogenesis and management of multiple organ dysfunction or failure in severe sepsis and septic shock. *Critical Care Clinics, 16,* 337-352.

Berry, B.E. (2002). Assessing tissue oxygenation. *Critical Care Nursing, 22,* 22-42.

Chaney, J.C., & Derdak, S. (2002). Minimally invasive hemodynamic monitoring for the intensivist: Current and emerging technology. *Critical Care Medicine, 30,* 2338-2345.

Copstead-Kirkhorn, L.E., & Banasik, J.L. (2005). *Pathophysiology* (3rd ed.). Philadelphia: W.B. Saunders.

Ely W., Kleinpell, R., & Goyette R. (2003). Systemic inflammatory response syndrome, multiple organ dysfunction syndrome, and recombinant human activated protein C: Important elements of severe sepsis. *American Journal of Critical Care 12,* 120-135.

Gawlinski, A., et al. (1999). Shock. In A. Gawlinski & D. Hamwi (Eds.). *Acute Care Nurse Practitioner Clinical Curriculum and Certification Review* (pp. 238-250). Philadelphia: W.B. Saunders.

Harrison's Online. Shock. Accessed January 5, 2003, from http://www.harrisonsonline.com.

Hochman, J.S., et al. (1999). Should we emergently revascularize occluded coronaries for cardiogenic shock? An international randomized trial of emergency PTCA/CABG-Trial design. *American Heart Journal, 137,* 313-321.

Hollenberg, S.M., Kavinsky, C.J., & Parrillo, J.E. (1999). Cardiogenic shock. *Annals of Internal Medicine, 131,* 47-59.

Jindal, N., Hollenberg, S.M., & Dellinger, R.P. (2000). Pharmacologic issues in the management of septic shock. *Critical Care Clinics, 16,* 233-249.

Kellum, J.A., & Pinsky, M.R. (2002). Use of vasopressor agents in critically ill patients. *Current Opinion in Critical Care, 8,* 236-241.

Kleinpell, R. (1998). Anaphylaxis: What you need to know to recognize, treat and prevent a life-threatening reaction. *Nursing98, 28,* 32hn1-32hn4.

Kruse, J.A., Fink, M.P., Carlson, R.W. (2003). *Saunders manual of critical care.* Philadelphia: W.B. Saunders.

Leach, R.M., & Treacher, D.F. (2002). The pulmonary physician in critical care: Oxygen delivery and consumption in the critically ill. *Thorax* 57, 170-177.

Niibori, K., Whitman, G.J. (1999). Shock. In P. Logan (Ed.). *Principles of practice for the acute care nurse practitioner.* Stamford, CT: Appleton & Lange, 237-246.

Schulman, C. (2002). End points of resuscitation: Choosing the right parameters to monitor. *Dimensions of Critical Care Nursing, 21,* 2-14.

Task Force of the American College of Critical Care Medicine. (1999). Practice parameters for hemodynamic support of sepsis in adult patients in sepsis. *Critical Care Medicine, 27,* 639-660.

Chapter 19

Sedation Management

Denise M. Meredith

1. **Define anxiety, agitation, and delirium. Describe implications these diagnoses may have in the acute care setting.**

Anxiety can be described as a subjective feeling of fear or apprehension of the unknown. Anxiety can be an emotional reaction to an unfamiliar experience such as a hospitalization. The anxious patient may display numerous different physical manifestations such as tachycardia, tachypnea, heart palpitations, tremors, and sweating. Anxiety can be displayed emotionally as fearfulness or tearfulness. Anxiety can interfere with concentration and sleep patterns ultimately resulting in feelings of fatigue and frustration.

Agitation is a bit harder to define and is more easily described by the outward appearance of the agitated patient. The agitated patient often exhibits a state of constant motion such as kicking, fidgeting, or climbing out of the bed. Agitation may result in pulling at lines and wires and dislodging tubes. The agitated patient may be disoriented and confused, conversing in a nonsensical pattern. If left untreated, the agitated patient can often become a physical threat to self or others.

Delirium is an acute and usually transient cognitive disorder. The pattern of delirium varies in intensity and duration. The delirious patient may present with alterations in cognition such as confusion and disorganized thinking. They are unable to concentrate or maintain attention. Agitation may accompany the clinical picture of delirium. There may be disturbances in perception manifesting as visual or auditory hallucinations. The delirious patient may experience disturbances in the sleep-wake cycle. The key clinical features of delirium are the abrupt onset and fluctuant course.

Anxiety, agitation, and delirium may have multiple implications for the patient in the acute care setting such as increased length of stay, increased cost, failure to participate in daily care plan, complications such as displacement of tubes or invasive lines, and increased time for mechanical ventilation.

2. **What diagnostic testing is indicated for the workup of the anxious, agitated, or delirious patient?**

Diagnostic Testing

Laboratory Studies

Complete blood count	Drug levels	Antinuclear antibody
Electrolytes	Toxicology screen	Thiamine
Blood urea nitrogen and creatinine	Urinalysis/urine culture	Folate
Ammonia	Liver function tests	Heavy metals
Arterial blood gas	Glucose	Human immunodeficiency virus
Blood culture	Erythrocyte sedimentation rate	Thyroid function tests

Other Studies

Computed tomography	Chest radiograph	Lumbar puncture
Magnetic resonance imaging	Electrocardiogram	Electroencephalogram

---

3. **List common causes of anxiety, agitation, and delirium.**
   - Reversible causes
     - Hypoxia*
     - Hypoglycemia
     - Hypotension*
     - Pain
     - Hospital-induced noxious stimuli (invasive tubes or devices, restraints, noise pollution, overstimulation or understimulation)
     - Sleep-wake cycle interruption
   - Metabolic derangements
     - Infection
     - Acid-base disturbance
     - Endocrine disorders
     - Electrolyte abnormalities
     - Vitamin deficiencies
     - Liver failure
     - Renal failure
     - Encephalopathy
   - Medications
     - Multiple medications including, but not limited to, various antibiotics, sedatives, steroids, cardioactive drugs, narcotics
   - Substance withdrawal
     - Alcohol
     - Steroids
     - Benzodiazepines
   - Intoxication
   - Head trauma

---

*Necessitates immediate intervention.

4. What are the indications for sedation?

Sedation is indicated when anxiety, agitation, or delirium interferes with the plan of care set for the individual patient. Resolution of agitation is a top priority due to the potentially dangerous complications that may result. Specific indications for sedation include facilitation of necessary therapies such as mechanical ventilation and certain intensive care unit (ICU) procedures. Sedation is indicated to induce sleep, improve patient comfort, and relieve anxiety. In the critically ill, sedation may be indicated to decrease oxygen consumption and is necessary during neuromuscular blockade to induce amnesia.

5. What are the pharmacological agents of choice for sedation?

To date, no one ideal drug has been identified for sedation. Very few randomized control trials have been performed to identify the optimal drug or combination of drugs best suited for this purpose. Drug therapy, when used appropriately, is an important component of agitation management. Numerous factors must be considered when choosing a particular regimen. Hemodynamic stability, pain control, the need for frequent awakening as in the neurological population, and time to extubation must guide the decision. The Society of Critical Care Medicine has made recommendations in the Clinical Practice Guidelines for the sustained use of sedatives and analgesics in the critically ill adult. The guidelines are developed by a panel of experts to guide decision making in this arena.

Opioids are the drug of choice for analgesia. When administered correctly, opioids can be titrated to maintain analgesia and can provide sedation at higher doses. It is important to ensure adequate pain relief in the acute care patient. Rule out pain as a cause for agitation before sedating the agitated patient. Fentanyl is favorable in the hemodynamically unstable patient. It does not cause histamine release, which can cause vasodilation, which potentiates low blood pressure.

Benzodiazepines are commonly used for sedation. They are highly lipophilic and therefore act quickly once in the system to produce a state of sedation. Intermittent dosing may be adequate, although a continuous infusion may be necessary to achieve a predetermined therapeutic goal. Always use the lowest effective dose to avoid oversedation or prolonged sedation. *Midazolam* is recommended for acute agitation. It is a short-acting benzodiazepine with rapid onset. Use cautiously in patients who are critically ill, are obese, have renal failure, or are nutritionally deplete with low albumin. Prolonged sedation has been documented in these populations. *Lorazepam* is recommended as an intermittent bolus drug as well as a continuous infusion. It is hemodynamically well tolerated alone or when used in combination with opioid therapy. There is no active metabolite. Return to baseline consciousness is easier to predict than with midazolam. *Diazepam,* like midazolam, has a rapid onset and when used as a bolus drug is also associated with rapid awakening. However, its usefulness as a sedation drug has diminished because long-acting active metabolites produce prolonged sedation with multiple dosing. Benzodiazepines should be discontinued slowly rather than abruptly to avoid withdrawal symptoms, especially when used for more than 2 weeks.

Propofol was originally indicated for the induction and maintenance of general anesthesia, but it is rapidly gaining popularity as a sedative in the ICU. Propofol is a central nervous system (CNS) depressant that binds to the chloride channel that contains the gamma aminobutyric acid receptor. Propofol rapidly produces a state of hypnosis. It can be associated with hypotension and bradycardia especially when used in the bolus dose form and is therefore not approved for bolus use in the ICU. An infusion can be initiated at 5 mcg/kg/min and titrated by increments of 5 to 10 mcg/kg/min every 5 to 10 minutes until the desired level of sedation is reached. It is easily titratable to produce varying levels of sedation. The use of propofol has merit in the neurological population in that wake-up times are predictable, allowing for frequent neurological evaluations. It is important to remember that propofol can be used for anxiolysis and amnesia. It has no analgesic properties. Patients sedated on a propofol infusion with a high probability of experiencing pain must be placed on pain medicine concurrently.

Delirium can cause extreme agitation. *Haloperidol* is the drug of choice to treat delirium. Haloperidol, a neuroleptic agent, blocks postsynaptic dopamine receptors in the brain. It is the least sedating of the antipsychotic medications available. Haloperidol is usually given via intermittent intravenous dosing. The dose is started small and titrated every 30 minutes until the desired effect is achieved. Once the agitation is controlled, a maintenance dose of haloperidol at 25% of the loading dose can be administered every 6 hours. A maximum dose of 40 mg/day should not be exceeded. When administered in higher doses, the QT interval must be monitored for prolongation. As with most neuroleptic drugs, haloperidol can have extrapyramidal effects. Patients on haloperidol therapy should be monitored for manifestations such as tardive dyskinesia, dystonia, akathisia, and pseudoparkinsonism.

6. What tools are available to monitor sedation therapy?

Continual evaluation and reassessment of the agitated patient and their response to therapeutic measures is of paramount importance. A predetermined therapeutic goal should be set and followed by the multidisciplinary team caring for the patient undergoing sedation measures. The Society of Critical Care Medicine has recently published guidelines that suggest that a protocol driven approach to sedation therapy with a subjective tool to monitor patient response to sedation therapy will enhance the treatment of agitation in the ICU as well as perhaps decrease costs, decrease length of stay, and decrease ventilator days as a result of less oversedation. Evaluation of the agitated-sedated patient is subjective, which results in multiple opinions and descriptions. To date, no gold standard has been recognized for the evaluation of the sedated patient.

Once a subjective tool is chosen to guide sedation therapy, it should be agreed upon by all disciplines caring for the acute care patient and used consistently to ensure an accurate description of the agitation-sedation level and uniform documentation.

The *Richmond Agitation-Sedation Scale (RASS)* was developed by a multi-disciplinary team at Virginia Commonwealth University at Richmond (see the following table). It is a 10-point scale with scores ranging from +4 to –5 to qualify levels of sedation and levels of anxiety and agitation in the adult ICU patient. A score of 0 denotes a calm and alert patient. The scale uses ability to maintain eye contact as a marker for titration of sedatives. The RASS score has high inter-rater reliability and validity in recent studies. It is easy to learn and perform, and allows for titration of sedative agents based on the patient's response to verbal and physical stimulation.

Richmond Agitation-Sedation Scale

Score	Term	Description
+4	Combative	Overtly combative or violent; immediate danger to staff
+3	Very agitated	Pulls on or removes tube(s) or catheter(s) or has aggressive behavior towards staff
+2	Agitated	Frequent non-purposeful movement or patient-ventilator dyssynchrony
+1	Restless	Anxious or apprehensive but movements not aggressive or vigorous
0	Alert and calm	
−1	Drowsy	Not fully alert but has sustained (>10 seconds) awakening, with eye contact, to voice
−2	Light sedation	Briefly (<10 seconds) awakens with eye contact to voice
−3	Moderate sedation	Any movement (but no eye contact) to voice
−4	Deep sedation	No response to voice, but any movement to physical stimulation
−5	Unarousable	No response to voice or physical stimulation

From Sessler, C.N., et al. (2002). The Richmond Agitation-Sedation Scale: Validity and reliability in adult intensive care unit patients. *American Journal of Respiratory Critical Care Medicine*, 166, 1338-1344.

The *Ramsay scale* is a 6-point scale with measures ranging from anxious to unresponsive (see the table on p. 228). This scale has been the most widely used ICU sedation scale despite any data supporting its reliability or validity for use in this population. The scale was not originally intended for clinical use.

Ramsay Scale

Score	Description
1	Anxious and agitated or restless or both
2	Cooperative, oriented, and tranquil
3	Responding to commands only
4	Brisk response to light glabellar tap
5	Sluggish response to light glabellar tap
6	No response to light glabellar tap

From Riker, R.R., Picard, J.T., & Gilles, F.L. (1999). Prospective evaluation of the Sedation-Agitation Scale for adult critically ill patients. *Critical Care Medicine, 27*(7), 1325-1329.

The *Riker Sedation-Agitation Scale (SAS)* is a 7-point sedation scale that has numerical values that coincide with sedation levels ranging from dangerous agitation to unarousable (see the following table). Similar to the RASS scale, the SAS allows for titration of sedation therapy to a predetermined sedation goal based on the patient's response to a stimulus, this time a noxious stimulus. This scale, too, has been studied to determine reliability and validity. The SAS scale was found to correlate well with the Ramsay scale, suggesting construct validity. It was found to be a reliable and valid tool to monitor and evaluate sedation levels when used by trained and experienced practitioners.

Riker Sedation-Agitation Scale (SAS)

Score	Term	Description
7	Dangerous agitation	Pulling at endotracheal tube, trying to remove catheters, climbing over bed rail, striking at staff, thrashing side-to-side
6	Very agitated	Does not calm despite frequent verbal reminding of limits; requires physical restraints, biting ET tube
5	Agitated	Anxious or mildly agitated, attempting to sit up, calms down to verbal instruction
4	Calm and cooperative	Calm, awakens easily, follows commands
3	Sedated	Difficult to arouse, awakens to verbal stimuli or gentle shaking but drifts off again, follows simple commands
2	Very sedated	Arouses to physical stimuli but does not communicate or follow commands, may move spontaneously
1	Unarousable	Minimal or no response to noxious stimuli, does not communicate of follow commands

From Riker, R.R., Picard, J.T., & Gilles, F.L. (1999). Prospective evaluation of the Sedation-Agitation Scale for adult critically ill patients. *Critical Care Medicine, 27*(7), 1325-1329.

The *Motor Activity Assessment Scale (MAAS)* is another tool developed by an intensivist to categorize the levels of sedation and agitation in the ICU patient (see the following table). Each score provides a detailed description of the patient's level of consciousness paired with simultaneous behaviors. The levels range from unarousable with no movement to dangerously agitated and climbing out of bed or striking at staff. In a recent study, the MAAS was found to be a reliable and valid tool to assess sedation level and guide titration of sedation therapy when used in a small cohort of surgical patients on ventilation in the ICU.

Motor Activity Assessment Scale (MAAS)

Score	Description	Definition
0	Unresponsive	Does not move with noxious stimulus
1	Responsive only to noxious stimuli	Opens eyes *OR* raises eyebrows *OR* turns head toward stimulus *OR* moves limbs with noxious stimulus
2	Responsive to touch or name	Opens eyes *OR* raises eyebrows *OR* turns head toward stimulus *OR* moves limbs when touched or name is spoken loudly
3	Calm and cooperative	No external stimulus is required to elicit movement *AND* patient is adjusting sheets or clothes purposefully and follows commands
4	Restless and cooperative	No external stimulus is required to elicit movement *AND* patient is picking at sheets or tubes *OR* uncovering self and follows commands
5	Agitated	No external stimulus is required to elicit movement *AND* attempting to sit up *OR* moves limbs out of bed *AND* does not consistently follow commands
6	Dangerously agitated, uncooperative	No external stimulus is required to elicit movement *AND* patient is pulling at tubes or catheters *OR* thrashing side to side *OR* striking at staff *OR* trying to climb out of bed *AND* does not calm down when asked

From Devlin, J.W., et al. (1999). Motor Activity Assessment Scale: A valid and reliable sedation scale for use with mechanically ventilated patients in an adult surgical intensive care unit. *Critical Care Medicine 27*(7), 1271-1275.

7. What are the goals or endpoints of sedation?

The goal or endpoint of sedation therapy is a calm patient who can be easily aroused and maintain a normal sleep-wake cycle. This goal should be established before initiating sedation therapy. It is important to consider the individual needs of each patient. Some patients require a much deeper level of sedation. For example, the patient with traumatic brain injury may require deep sedation to aid in the management of intracranial hypertension. It is important to tailor the sedation plan according to which patient population is being treated. The patient's response to sedation therapy should be monitored at regular intervals and documented uniformly by all involved in the care of the patient to ensure optimal delivery of sedation therapy.

8. What is ICU psychosis?

ICU psychosis is a state of delirium that can be brought on by the stressful environment of the ICU. Factors such as invasive monitoring, overstimulation, noise pollution, constant ambient lighting, disruption of sleep-wake cycles, immobility, and loss of independence may lead to a state of cognitive disturbance resulting in agitated behavior. It is important to rule out other causes of delirium before labeling the agitated patient as having "ICU psychosis." Therapy of choice is haloperidol. Benzodiazepines may be used for acute episodes of agitation. Promoting restful periods and normal sleep-wake cycles may improve this disorder.

9. What is alcohol withdrawal syndrome? How is it treated?

Alcohol withdrawal syndrome results from a sudden cessation of alcohol ingestion, especially after the patient consumes large quantities on a regular basis. Alcohol withdrawal can present as mild (anxiety, irritability) to full blown delirium tremens (DTs). DTs usually present within 24 to 72 hours of the last drink. It can be a life-threatening situation. The patient may experience severe agitation, confusion, hallucinations, tachycardia, hypertension, and in the most serious cases, seizures. Benzodiazepines are the treatment of choice to depress CNS hyperactivity. In severe cases, a continuous infusion is necessary to gain control of the agitated patient. Clonidine may be added to lower severe hypertension and may also enhance the sedative effect of the benzodiazepines. Once sedation is achieved, the benzodiazepine dose should be tapered by 20% per day until withdrawal symptoms subside.

Key Points

- Anxiety, agitation, and delirium may have multiple implications for the patient in the acute care setting such as increased length of stay, increased cost, failure to participate in daily care plan, complications such as displacement of tubes or invasive lines, and increased time for mechanical ventilation.

- The following causes of agitation are life threatening and necessitate immediate intervention:
  - Reversible causes
    - Hypoxia
    - Hypoglycemia
    - Hypotension

- Ensure adequate pain control before treating agitation pharmacologically.

- Sedation is indicated when anxiety, agitation, or delirium interferes with the plan of care set for the individual patient. Resolution of agitation is a top priority because of the potentially dangerous complications that may result.

Key Points *continued*

- A protocol driven approach to sedation therapy with a subjective tool to monitor patient response to sedation therapy enhances the treatment of agitation in the ICU as well as perhaps decreasing costs, length of stay, and ventilator days because there is less oversedation.

- Continual evaluation and reassessment of the agitated patient and the patient's response to therapeutic measures is of paramount importance. Once a subjective tool is chosen to guide sedation therapy, it should be agreed upon by all disciplines caring for the acute care patient and used consistently to ensure an accurate description of the agitation-sedation level and uniform documentation.

Internet Resources

Veterans Health Administration: National Anesthesia Service: JCAHO Information: www.anesthesia.med.va.gov/anesthesia/page.cfm?pg=7

American Society of Anesthesiologists Newsletter: Sedation and the Need for Anesthesia Personnel: www.asahq.org/Newsletters/2002/3_02/pm302.htm

American Journal of Critical Care: Critical Care Management of Sedation: Sedating Critically Ill Patients: Factors Affecting Nurses' Delivery of Sedative Therapy: www.aacn.org/AACN/jrnlajcc.nsf/GetArticle/ArticleFour103?OpenDocument

Bibliography

Bower, C.T., & Vanderheyden, B.A. (2002). Analgesia, sedation, and neuromuscular blockade in the trauma patient. In K.A. McQuillan, et al. (Eds.), *Trauma nursing: From resuscitation through rehabilitation* (pp. 324-365). Philadelphia: W.B. Saunders.

Clark, S. (1999). Mental health disorders. In A. Gawlinski & D. Hamwi (Eds.), *Acute care nurse practitioner clinical curriculum and certification review* (pp. 859-904). Philadelphia: W.B. Saunders.

Cohen, I., et al. (2002). The management of the agitated ICU patient: A continuing education program sponsored jointly by the Postgraduate Institute for Medicine and Health Management Solutions, Inc. *Critical Care Medicine 30* (1; Suppl.), S97-S123.

Devlin, J.W., et al. (1999). Motor Activity Assessment Scale: A valid and reliable sedation scale for use with mechanically ventilated patients in an adult surgical intensive care unit. *Critical Care Medicine 27*(7), 1271-1275.

Eisendrath, S.J., & Lictmacher, J.E. (1999). Psychiatric disorders. In L.M. Tierney, S.J. McPhee, & M.A. Papadakis (Eds.), *Current medical diagnosis and treatment* (pp. 990-1048). Stamford, CT: Appleton & Lange.

Jacobi, J., et al. (2003). Clinical practice guidelines for the sustained use of sedatives and analgesics in the critically ill adult. *Critical Care Medicine 30*(1), 119-140.

Krupnick, S.L. (1999). The hospitalized patient's psychological response to illness. In P. Logan (Ed.), *Principles of practice for the acute care nurse practitioner* (pp. 1275-1310). Stamford, CT: Appleton & Lange.

Marino, P. (1998). Analgesia and sedation. In *The ICU Book* (2nd ed., pp. 121-139). Baltimore: Williams & Wilkins.

Neligan, P., et al. (2003). *Analgesia and sedation in the SICU: Surgical critical care clinical practice guidelines.* Unpublished manuscript, University of Pennsylvania Medical Center/Hospital of the University of Pennsylvania Department of Surgery.

Ostermann, M.E., et al. (2000). Sedation in the intensive care unit: A systematic review. *Journal of the American Medical Association 283*(11), 1451-1459.

Rabow, M.W., & Brody, R.V. (1999). Care at the end of life. In L.M. Tierney, S.J. McPhee, & M.A. Papadakis (Eds.), *Current medical diagnosis and treatment* (pp. 104-115). Stamford, CT: Appleton & Lange.

Riker, R.R., Picard, J.T., & Gilles, F.L. (1999). Prospective evaluation of the Sedation-Agitation Scale for adult critically ill patients. *Critical Care Medicine, 27*(7), 1325-1329.

Sessler, C.N., et al. (2002). The Richmond Agitation-Sedation Scale: Validity and reliability in adult intensive care unit patients. *American Journal of Respiratory Critical Care Medicine, 166,* 1338-1344.

Thomas, M. (1992). Anxiety and agitation in the ICU. In P.E. Parsons, & J.P. Wiener-Kronish (Eds.), *Critical care secrets* (pp. 432-437). Philadelphia: Hanley & Belfus.

Thomas, M. (1992). Delirium. In P.E. Parsons, & J.P. Wiener-Kronish (Eds.), *Critical care secrets* (pp. 426-431). Philadelphia: Hanley & Belfus.

Wesley, E.E., et al. (2003). Monitoring sedation status over time in ICU patients: Reliability and validity of the Richmond Agitation-Sedation Scale (RASS). *Journal of the American Medical Association, 289*(22), 2983-2991.

Chapter 20

Pain Management

Catherine Cristofalo

1. What are the JCAHO standards for pain management?

- Recognize the right of patients to appropriate assessment and management of pain.
- Assess the existence, nature, and intensity of pain in all patients.
- Record the results to facilitate regular assessment and follow-up.
- Determine and ensure staff competency in pain assessment and management.
- Establish policies and procedures to support the prescription of effective pain management.
- Educate patients and families about effective pain management.
- Address patient needs for symptom management in the discharge planning process.

2. What constitutes acute pain versus chronic pain?

Acute pain is often associated with injury or acute illness and resolves over time, disappearing when the healing process is complete. Signs of acute pain include tachypnea, tachycardia, pallor, and other symptoms associated with activation of the autonomic nervous system. Acute pain is often localized.

Chronic pain is usually defined as pain lasting greater than 1 month beyond disease or injury or lasting greater than 3 months in the absence of an inciting event. Chronic pain may not be associated with a specific injury and may be poorly localized. Autonomic nervous system activation symptoms are usually not present, because the body adapts over time.

Psychological symptoms, such as depression and anger, frequently coincide with chronic pain. Malignant or cancer pain often has characteristics of both types of pain (see the box on p. 234).

3. How are pain signals transmitted?

Peripheral nerves are made up of three types: primary sensory afferents, motor neurons, and sympathetic postganglionic neurons. The primary sensory afferent nerves are further delineated in regard to feeling the pain sensation. The two main types of peripheral nerves involved in the transmission of pain are A delta

Characteristics of Acute and Chronic Pain

Acute Pain
Acute onset
Tachypnea
Tachycardia
Diaphoresis
Pallor
Often localized
Limited duration

Chronic Pain
Onset insidious
Duration >1 month
Poorly localized
Absence of sympathetic responses
Associated psychological symptoms

fibers (myelinated) and C fibers (unmyelinated). These fibers innervate the skin, visceral, and somatic structures. *A Delta fibers* are fast-transmitting fibers, and *C fibers* are slow-transmitting fibers. The largest fibers, called beta fibers, are also primary afferent fibers. These fibers enable the feeling of light touch. They do not typically produce pain, but in syndromes such as trigeminal neuralgia and other neuropathic syndromes, they can be responsible for allodynia, which is a normally painless sensation that can be perceived as excruciating (see the figure below).

It is thought that the main neurotransmitters secreted to produce pain are glutamate and *substance P.*

The two receptors for these two substances are NMDA (*N*-methyl-D-aspartate) and AMPA (alpha-amino-3-hydroxy-5-methyl-4-isoxazolepropionic acid). Substance P is associated with acute pain, whereas glutamate and NMDA receptors are associated with chronic pain, especially neuropathic pain. Other neurotransmitters involved include 5-HT or serotonin, prostaglandins,

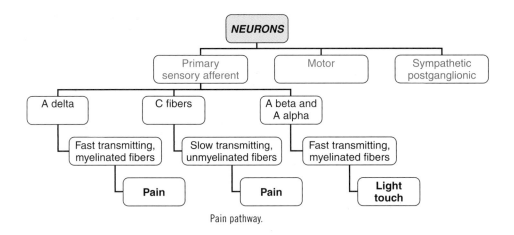

Pain pathway.

norepinephrine, histamine, leukotrienes, gamma aminobutyric acid (GABA), and bradykinin. This is a simplified explanation, although it is important to have some familiarity with these terms in order to understand pain treatment, specifically the pharmacological therapies (see the following box).

Pain Neurotransmitters

- Glutamate
- Substance P
- 5-HT
- Prostaglandins
- Norepinephrine
- Histamine
- Leukotrienes
- Gamma aminobutyric acid
- Bradykinin
- Potassium ions
- Receptors
- NMDA
- AMPA
- Neurokinin–1

AMPA, Alpha-amino-3-hydroxy-5-methyl-4-isoxazolepropionic acid; NMDA, N-methyl-ᴅ-aspartate.

4. What are endogenous opioids?

Endogenous opioids are the naturally occurring pain relievers that are released in response to pain. They are endorphins, enkephalins, and dynorphins.

5. What are the three main analgesic receptors?

The three main analgesic receptors are the mu, kappa, and sigma receptors. These have an affinity for pure opioid agonists. These receptors are present throughout the central nervous system and in peripheral tissues. They are the receptors for both endogenous endorphins and opioid medications. For example, morphine and its derivative medications bind to the mu receptor. Binding to these receptor sites decreases the transmission of pain-producing neurotransmitters, especially of substance P, through A delta and C fibers. The following table lists the effects produced when binding occurs on certain receptor sites.

Analgesic Receptors

Mu	Kappa	Sigma
Analgesia	Analgesia	Analgesia
Euphoria	Sedation	
Sedation		
Respiratory depression		

6. **How are the different types of pain classified in relation to anatomical origin?**

- *Somatic pain:* Nociceptors are activated in the cutaneous and the subcutaneous tissues, as well as the deep tissues including vascular, muscle, bone, and connective tissues. It is usually well localized.
- *Visceral pain:* Nociceptors are activated in the organs and linings of the body cavities. The pain is often poorly differentiated and may be referred.
- *Neuropathic pain:* Nociceptors are activated in the central nervous system, spinal cord, or peripheral nerves.

7. **What are the essential components for a thorough pain assessment?**

Assessment of pain should begin with *onset and duration*. It is important to further identify whether the symptoms occurred suddenly or insidiously, and whether there was a specific event that precipitated the pain. Inquire about the location of pain including the distribution or radiating quality. Does it occur in a stocking-glove pattern such as in diabetic neuropathy or is it dermatomal, such as in herpes zoster or radiculopathy? It can be helpful to have the patient draw on a preprinted body diagram a subjective picture of where the pain occurs.

Be sure to inquire about pain *descriptors*, such as "burning," "throbbing," "aching," or "stabbing." These descriptors can be useful in identifying the type of pain. For example, burning pain is often neuropathic in nature and cramping or gnawing pain may be visceral.

Factors that *exacerbate or alleviate* pain should be identified.

Severity of pain should be established. Pain scales are helpful, such as the numeric scales that rate pain from 0 to 10, the Visual Analogue Scale, descriptive word scales, and face or picture rating scales, which are often useful in pediatric patients. New pain scales are being developed to incorporate all or some of these models in one scale.

Pain diaries are also helpful in following pain and efficacy of intervention over time.

A complete history and physical examination is in order when diagnosing pain syndromes. Allergies should be documented. Past medical, family, and social histories aid in the differential diagnosis.

8. **What differential diagnoses should be considered when a patient complains of pain?**

A useful mnemonic that includes all of the differential diagnoses is VINDICATE (see the box on p. 237).

Differentiating Pain: Pain Mnemonic

V: Viral or infectious in etiology, such as AIDS-related pain or post-herpetic neuralgia after herpes zoster infection or even after acute bacterial, viral, or fungal infections

I: Inflammation, such as in arthropathies, radiculopathies, or other autoimmune or rheumatologic disorders

N: Neoplasm

D: Degenerative disorders, such as connective tissue disorders

I: Ischemic disease, such as in mesenteric ischemia or peripheral vascular insufficiency

C: Congenital disorders associated with altered neurological development

A: Autoimmune disorders, which can be responsible for neuropathic type pain

T: Trauma

E: Endocrine or metabolic, such as diabetic neuropathy

---

9. **What is the best way to treat breakthrough pain?**

Breakthrough medication is short-acting medication for patients with pain exacerbation, or episodic or incident pain. Many of these short-acting medications are combined with either acetaminophen or aspirin, providing a synergistic effect. The limitation to this method is that both of these medications have dosing limitations: acetaminophen in high doses is hepatotoxic; aspirin (ASA) causes gastrointestinal upset and bleeding, and nonsteroid anti-inflammatory drugs (NSAIDs) cause gastrointestinal side effects as well as renal toxicity. Examples include oxycodone with acetaminophen (Percocet), hydrocodone with acetaminophen (Vicodin), hydrocodone with ibuprofen (Vicoprofen), oxycodone with ASA (Percodan), propoxyphene with Tylenol (Darvocet), and acetaminophen with codeine.

10. **What are examples of adjuvant agents?**

Adjuvant medications should be used when treating pain, especially neuropathic pain. Examples of adjuvant medications are tricyclic antidepressants, anticonvulsants, benzodiazepines, antihistamines, and steroids. Topical preparations are either anesthetic (e.g., EMLA cream or Lidoderm Patch) or nonanesthetic (e.g., capsaicin cream). Adjuvants are essential in treating neuropathic pain and can be useful also in treating most chronic pain syndromes.

11. **What should be considered when treating mild pain?**

Nonopioid medications should be used when treating mild pain. These include NSAIDs, acetaminophen, and COX-2 inhibitors. As mentioned earlier, these medications do have side effects and should be used with caution. COX-2 inhibitors are reported to provide less gastrointestinal irritation than traditional NSAIDs, but there is no benefit in regard to renal toxicity. In addition, COX-2 inhibitors have been associated with an increased risk of cardiovascular complications.

12. What are the recommendations of the World Health Organization for the treatment of cancer pain?

In 1986 the World Health Organization (WHO) issued a statement regarding the treatment of cancer pain. They created an analgesic three-step ladder:
- Step One: Use nonopioid analgesic such as acetaminophen or NSAID with or without adjuvant medication.
- Step Two: If pain increases or persists, use mild opioid with or without nonopioid or adjuvant.
- Step Three: If pain increases or persists, use a stronger opioid with or without nonopioid or adjuvant with breakthrough medication as needed.

Strong opioids are morphine, intravenous (IV) Demerol, Dilaudid, fentanyl, and methadone.

13. Why is Demerol not a good choice for pain medication?

Demerol has a metabolite, normeperidine, which is neurotoxic. It can produce symptoms such as seizures, myoclonus, tremors, and anxiety as it accumulates. Oral Demerol has only one fourth of the analgesic effectiveness of parenteral doses but has equal metabolite accumulation. As it is renally excreted, it is even more dangerous in the renally compromised population.

14. What are available long-acting opioid preparations?

Long-acting opioids are useful in the treatment of chronic pain for a variety of reasons, but mostly to keep a steady state of pain relief. Available preparations include sustained-release morphine, which is available in generic form, but which is known also as Kadian, Avinza, and Morphine (MS) Contin. Sustained-release oxycodone (OxyContin) is also an effective long-acting medication. These preparations have a tendency to be abused. This is done by disabling the time-release structure of the pill by chewing it, crushing it, or dissolving it into liquid form and then eating, snorting, or injecting the compound. Methadone, which is not in sustained-release form, is inherently long acting with a half-life of approximately 24 to 36 hours. Fentanyl is a very short-acting opioid with almost no metabolite accumulation. Duragesic is a fentanyl-impregnated patch, which makes it an option for 24-hour pain coverage. The transdermal fentanyl patch is usually changed every 72 hours, but some patients change the patch every 48 hours to obtain continuous relief. The dosing of the patch is in micrograms released per hour.

Sustained-relief morphine and oxycodone are dosed every 12 hours routinely, but they may be given every 8 hours. This is helpful to achieve smaller dose increases and better 24-hour coverage in some patients.

15. What is patient-controlled analgesia (PCA) and how is it used?

PCA is frequently used in both hospitalized cancer pain patients and post-surgical patients. PCA may be given either intravenously or epidurally. The most common medications used are morphine, hydromorphone, and fentanyl. Epidural preparations are usually mixed with a local anesthetic for regional anesthesia. Several infusion settings can be chosen. Some clinicians give a loading dose for initial analgesia. One may opt to give patients a basal rate, which is a continuous medication infusion. This should be used with much caution, especially in older adults, because it can result in oversedation. The PCA dose is the setting of the amount of medication the patient will receive intermittently. To avoid overdose, a lockout time is set in minutes. Furthermore, a 1- or 4-hour maximum dose is set.

The benefit of PCA is that the patient receives the medication as soon as he or she feels pain. It is also helpful to titrate doses based on need. The pump keeps a record of how many times the patient attempted to get the medication and how many times he or she actually received it. PCA is also safe in that the medication is delivered in small short-acting doses, so it is difficult for one to become severely oversedated. On the other hand, if a patient falls asleep or is unable to push the button, the patient is left without medication during that time and may experience severe pain.

16. What are the basic principles behind opioid conversion?

Understanding the need for dose conversion when changing opioids is the most important step. There are several charts for conversions that may be used as guides, but all differ to some degree. Some individuals perform conversions based on the relationship of the drug to morphine, the opioid "gold standard." In other words, if the drug conversion to morphine is known, then first convert the drug to morphine and then to the drug selected. For example, if converting from fentanyl to oxycodone, first convert fentanyl to morphine, which is about 1000 times less potent, and then convert the morphine dose to oxycodone. For example, 100 micrograms of IV fentanyl equals 10 mg of IV morphine, which equals 20 to 30 mg of oral oxycodone. More practically, if a patient requires 30 mg of IV morphine over 24 hours and it is desired to switch to an oral preparation such as oxycodone with acetaminophen (Percocet), assume the patient needs 60 to 80 mg of oxycodone in 24 hours. Then, divide the dose into appropriate dosing intervals, which for Percocet is approximately every 4 hours. This patient will need approximately two 5 mg Percocet every 4 hours.

Other factors to consider during drug conversion are that the conversion may differ in high doses and that dosing schedules and degree of accumulation of certain medications also differ. Furthermore, conversion is also necessary in changing routes of delivery, such as intravenous to oral, because bioavailability is variable (see the box on p. 240).

17. When is it desirable to rotate opioids?

Opioid rotation is often helpful when doses escalate because of tolerance. It has become apparent that different opioids bind to many different subreceptors, allowing lower dosing with a change in the particular opioid.

> ## Opioid Equianalgesia
>
> | | |
> |---|---|
> | Morphine IV: 10 mg | Oxycodone PO: 20 to 30 mg |
> | Morphine PO: 30 mg | Methadone IV: 10 mg |
> | Fentanyl IV: 0.1 mg | Methadone PO: 20 mg |
> | Hydromorphone IV: 1.5 mg | Hydrocodone PO: 30 mg |
> | Hydromorphone PO: 7.5 mg | Codeine PO: 180 mg |

18. What is Ultram (tramadol)?

Ultram is a nonscheduled synthetic analogue of codeine, although it has a low affinity for the mu receptor and is only partially reversed with the use of naloxone (Narcan). It is a centrally acting analgesic, in which the mechanism of action is not entirely understood. It does, however, have effects on norepinephrine and serotonin. It can result in serotonin syndrome when used concomitantly with some antidepressants. Ultram has a ceiling effect as well, unlike opioids, meaning that beyond a certain dose there is no increase in pain relief. High doses can result in seizures and patients with a history of seizure disorders should avoid this medication.

19. What are the most common opioid side effects?

Urinary retention, nausea, constipation, and sedation are common side effects of opioids. Frequently, in the postoperative period, vomiting occurs as the chemoreceptor trigger zone is stimulated. Orthostasis and hypotension may occur as the vasomotor center becomes depressed. There is decreased gastric acid secretion and biliary tract contraction. Confusion often occurs in older adults. Dysphoria may occur when people do not have pain. Respiratory depression is the most serious sign of overmedication and is dose related. Cough suppression occurs.

Narcotic overdose can be reversed with naloxone, a pure opioid receptor antagonist. Early signs of overmedication with narcotics may be reflected by myosis of the pupil. Constipation and myosis are two side effects that do not disappear with opioid tolerance, unlike the other side effects, which are rarely seen in the opioid-tolerant patient. Therefore it is essential to give patients on opioids stool softeners, such as Senokot or Colace.

20. How does one recognize opioid withdrawal?

Withdrawal from opioids may be seen in anyone who has taken opioids for as long as 2 weeks and abruptly stops the opioid. Withdrawal can occur at different times depending on the half-life of the drug given. For example, a patient who takes oxycodone over a long period will have symptoms of withdrawal before a patient who stops methadone, which is very long acting.

Signs of withdrawal include the following:
- Neurological excitability, which can be manifested as agitation, tremors, irritability, seizures, hyperreflexia, increased muscle tone, and tachypnea. In pediatric patients, it may manifest as inability to suck and inconsolable crying.
- Gastrointestinal effects include abdominal cramping, diarrhea, and vomiting
- Autonomic hyperactivity includes tachycardia, diaphoresis, itching, dilated pupils, and fever.

There are several important concepts to remember about withdrawal:
- First, do not undermedicate the opioid-tolerant patient during a stressful event such as hospitalization or surgery.
- Second, be careful when using opioid antagonists such as naloxone, because these medications can precipitate the symptoms of withdrawal.
- Third, the cure for withdrawal symptoms is opioid. Benzodiazepines, such as clonazepam, are also helpful, in addition to alpha-2 receptor agonists such as clonidine.
- Tapering opioids is essential for discontinuation. One method is to give the patient one half of the previous daily dose for the first 2 days and reduce by 25% every 2 days. When the minimum dose is reached, use it for 2 days and then discontinue. Patients taking very large doses who have other dependency issues may need a slower wean. Methadone is also frequently used for weaning, starting at one fourth of the equianalgesic dose to start.

21. What is neuropathic pain and how is it treated?

Neuropathic pain occurs after a nerve insult or injury and the nerve fibers discharge inappropriately. Anticonvulsants are used to treat neuropathic pain, because the mechanism of action is inhibition of sodium-gated channels and the potentiation of GABA-ergic receptors. Examples are carbamazepine (Tegretol) and gabapentin (Neurontin). Some medications such as carbapentin can be hepatotoxic; therefore liver function must be monitored. Tricyclic antidepressants are useful in the treatment of neuropathic type pain. Caution must be observed with these medications because they may result in dysrhythmias and are lethal with overdose. Nortriptyline and amitriptyline are the most commonly used. Combinations of these medications with an opioid, anti-inflammatory, or a muscle relaxer are often helpful in neuropathic syndromes. Medications with NMDA receptor blockade, such as methadone, are also helpful. Interventional pain management with injection therapy to desensitize nerves and decrease inflammation around the nerves is also helpful. Examples are local nerve blocks or sympathetic chain blocks, as well as epidural injections. Spinal cord stimulators may also be useful.

22. **What is the common differential diagnosis with neuropathic pain?**
    - Post-herpetic neuralgia
    - Sciatica or other spinal etiologies
    - Nerve injuries due to trauma or surgery
    - Reflex sympathetic dystrophy
    - Central pain syndromes
    - Trigeminal neuralgia
    - Diabetic or peripheral neuropathy

23. **What is the probable diagnosis for a patient, who presents with a painful, edematous, discolored extremity after casting for a lower extremity fracture?**

    The most likely diagnosis is complex regional pain syndrome (CRPS), which frequently occurs in the limbs, either unilaterally or bilaterally, and may occur in the neck area. The most common causes are fracture, tight casting, surgical procedure, or trauma, but the cause of many cases of CRPS is unknown. The general pathogenesis is sympathetic system overactivation, resulting in ischemia.

    CRPS is an incapacitating syndrome that often is left to progress because of misdiagnosis. There are two types, although treatment is the same. Type one is reflex sympathetic dystrophy (RSD) and type two is causalgia. In causalgia there is a known nerve injury.

24. **What common symptoms are associated with CRPS?**
    - Edema
    - Hyperalgesias
    - Allodynia
    - Changes in skin color
    - Atrophy and excessive sweating in the affected area
    - In the late stages, cyanosis of the affected area

25. **How is CRPS diagnosed?**

    Diagnosis is made mainly by physical examination. Triple-phase bone scan shows decreased uptake of radioactive nucleotide in the affected area, because blood flow to the bone is diminished. However, disuse alone can cause this finding, so it is not necessarily specific for diagnosis.

26. **What is the treatment of CRPS?**

    Treatment is multifactorial and includes sympathetic nerve blocks or chemical or neuroablation for permanent sympathetic nerve lysis to improve blood flow. Pharmacology may include combinations such as alpha-2 agonists like clonidine, as well as opioids, tricyclic antidepressants or selective serotonin reuptake inhibitors, anti-inflammatories, and muscle relaxers. Desensitization to pain is essential as is stimulation or use of the limb or area to help restore blood flow. A good physical therapy program is essential as well is treatment of other comorbidities such as depression, sleep deprivation, and poor nutrition.

27. **What is the difference between tolerance, physical dependence, psychological dependence, addiction, and pseudoaddiction?**

- Tolerance occurs with continued use of a drug, resulting in decreased efficacy and need for dose increases to obtain the same efficacy.
- Physical dependence is the physiological need for the drug after consuming it over a period of time. Abrupt cessation causes withdrawal.
- Psychological dependence is an emotional need for the drug for either its positive effects or to avoid the negative effects associated with not taking the drug.
- Addiction is an uncontrollable use of the drug that can result in physical, psychological, economic, legal, or social harm to the user or others.
- Pseudoaddiction can result if an individual's pain is not adequately managed, causing him or her to revert to deviant or drug-seeking behaviors.

These syndromes are often difficult to diagnose and may require evaluation by a pain specialist or mental health professional.

28. **What alternative or mind-body therapies are helpful for pain management?**

This is a rapidly expanding field, which is most useful in chronic pain management. Some examples of alternative therapies follow:
- Biofeedback
- Yoga
- Massage therapy
- Reflexology
- Pain diaries
- Acupuncture
- Hypnosis
- Aromatherapy
- Meditation
- Transcutaneous electrical nerve stimulation
- Therapeutic touch

These therapies are becoming more and more available. Alternative therapies are not always used in place of conventional pain management with medication, but they are useful in reducing medication requirements, promoting better mental health, and empowering the pain patient.

29. Why is a multidisciplinary approach to pain management so important?

Chronic pain affects every aspect of an individual's life and is best managed by a multidisciplinary approach, with each specialist contributing strategies in his or her area of expertise. After initial consultation with a pain specialist, chronic pain sufferers should see a mental health professional for coping and management of other comorbid pathologies that are often present, such as depression and addiction. Rehabilitation specialists help in desensitization as well as in treatment of the inciting pathology in cases such as low back pain. Chronic pain patients must deal with social issues as well, because frequently they are unable to work, making social workers helpful in sorting out social issues.

30. What is the concept of central sensitization?

Central sensitization occurs after prolonged stimulation of the nerves, in the presence of tissue injury or damage. The threshold for activating nociceptors is lowered. Bradykinin, leukotrienes, and prostaglandins play a role in this phenomenon. When a tissue becomes sensitized, hyperalgesias or pain with temperature variations and allodynia, which is pain invoked by otherwise non-painful stimuli, frequently occur. Again, adequate pain relievers are essential for reversal. Repeated nerve blocks and physical therapy are also mainstays of treatment.

🔑 Key Points

- Pain standards have been set by JCAHO. It is now considered the fifth vital sign. Institutions and health care professionals will be held accountable to ensure the proper treatment of pain.
- A multidisciplinary approach to pain management should be used for better outcomes.
- Different types of pain should be managed using specific treatment modalities for that type of pain.

Internet Resources

Hospice.net: Pain:
www.hospicenet.org/html/what_is_pain.html

American Pain Society:
www.ampainsoc.org

Pain.com:
www.pain.com

Bibliography

American Pain Society. (1999). *Principles of analgesic use in the treatment of acute pain and cancer pain* (4th ed.). Glenview, IL: Author.

Backonja, M., & Galer, B. (1998). Neuropathic pain syndromes. *Neurologic Clinics, 16*(4), 775-789.

Bennett, G. (1998). Neuropathic pain: New insights, new interventions. *Hospital Practice, 33*(10), 95-110.

Besson, J. (1999). The neurobiology of pain. *The Lancet, 353*(9164), 1610-1615.

Buck, M. (2000). Managing iatrogenic opioid dependence with methadone. *Pediatric Pharmacotherapy, 6*(7). Retrieved January 15, 2005, from www.medscape.com.

Gavrin, J. (1999). New challenges in anesthesia: New practice opportunities. *Anesthesia Clinics of North America, 17*(2), 467-477.

Logan, P. (1999). Principles of practice for the acute care nurse practitioner. Stamford, CT: Appleton & Lange.

Schurmann, M., et al. (2001). Clinical and physiologic evaluation of stellate ganglion blockade for complex regional pain syndrome type I. *The Clinical Journal of Pain, 17*(1), 94-100.

Wesselmann, U., & Srinivasa, R. (1997). Pain: Nociceptive and neuropathic mechanisms. *Anesthesiology Clinics of North America, 15*(2), 407-428.

Woolf, C., & Max, M. (2001). Mechanism based pain diagnosis: Issues for analgesic drug development. *Anesthesiology, 95*(1), 241-249.

Woolf, C., & Mannion, R. (1999). Neuropathic pain: Etiology, symptoms, mechanism and management. Lancet, *353*(9168), 1959-1964.

World Health Organization. (1996). Cancer pain relief: with a guide to opioid availability (2nd ed.). Geneva, Author.

Chapter 21

Ventilator Management

Wendy Stevens

1. How is respiratory failure defined?

- Inability to maintain oxygen uptake and CO_2 clearance as defined by PaO_2, PCO_2, and pH levels.
- PaO_2 below normal range for patient's age (hypoxemic respiratory failure)
- $PaCO_2$ >50 and rising (hypercapnic failure)
- PH ≤7.25

2. Identify causes of respiratory failure.

The causes of respiratory failure are listed in the box on p. 248.

3. What manifestations are associated with hypoxia?

MILD TO MODERATE EFFECTS (EARLY MANIFESTATIONS)
- Neurological: restlessness, headaches, mental status changes
- Cardiovascular: tachycardia, mild hypertension
- Respiratory: tachypnea, dyspnea
- Skin: paleness

SEVERE EFFECTS (LATE MANIFESTATIONS)
- Neurological: somnolence, tunneled or blurred vision, slow reaction time, coma
- Cardiovascular: tachycardia developing into bradycardia, dysrhythmias, hypotension
- Respiratory: tachypnea, dyspnea
- Skin: cyanosis

4. What manifestations are associated with hypercapnia?

MILD TO MODERATE EFFECTS
- Neurological: drowsiness, headaches, diaphoresis
- Cardiovascular: tachycardia, mild hypertension
- Respiratory: tachypnea, dyspnea
- Skin: reddened

(Continued on p. 249)

Causes of Respiratory Failure

Disorders of the Central Nervous System

Depressant drugs
- Barbiturates
- Sedatives
- General anesthetics
- Narcotics

Brain or brainstem lesions
- Stroke
- Trauma to head or neck
- Cerebral hemorrhage
- Tumors
- Spinal cord injury

Hypothyroidism

Sleep apnea

Inappropriate oxygen therapy

Disorders of Neuromuscular Function

Paralytic disorders
- Myasthenia gravis
- Tetanus
- Botulism
- Guillain-Barré syndrome
- Poliomyelitis
- Muscular dystrophy
- Amyotrophic lateral sclerosis

Paralytic drugs

Drugs affecting neuromuscular transmission
- Aminoglycoside antibiotics
- Long-term corticosteroids
- Calcium channel blockers

Impaired muscle function
- Fatigue
- Electrolyte imbalances
- Malnutrition
- Peripheral nerve disorders
- Atrophy

Disorders in Increased Work of Breathing

Pleural space lesions
- Effusions
- Hemothorax
- Empyema
- Pneumothorax

Chest wall abnormalities
- Flail chest
- Rib fracture
- Obesity
- Kyphoscoliosis

Increased airway resistance
- Secretions
- Mucosal edema
- Bronchoconstriction
- Foreign body
- Inflammation (e.g., asthma, croup, bronchitis, acute epiglottitis)

Lung tissue involvement
- Acute respiratory distress syndrome
- Cardiogenic pulmonary edema
- Idiopathic pulmonary fibrosis
- Aspiration

Pulmonary vascular problems
- Pulmonary embolism
- Pulmonary vascular damage

Dynamic hyperinflation or air trapping

SEVERE EFFECTS
- Neurological: hallucinations, convulsions, coma
- Cardiovascular: hypotension
- Respiratory: bradypnea

5. What are the standard indications for mechanical ventilation?

- Apnea
- Acute respiratory failure
- Impending respiratory failure with hypoxemia or respiratory acidosis despite treatment
- Anesthesia-induced hypoventilation

6. What are the two types of mechanical ventilation?

VOLUME VENTILATION
- A preset volume is delivered during the mandatory breath.
- Assist control and spontaneous intermittent mechanical ventilation (SIMV) are the ventilator modes.
- Overdistention of alveoli is one of the main risks.

PRESSURE VENTILATION
- With preset pressure, the volume delivered varies depending on lung characteristics.
- IMV/SIMV are the ventilator modes.
- Variability of volume delivered is one of the main risks.

7. What are the most common initial ventilator settings?

- *Rate:* 14 to 20
- *Positive end-expiratory pressure (PEEP):* 5 cm H_2O to close to physiological intrinsic PEEP
- *Tidal volume (V_t):* 8 mL/kg if not underlying pulmonary issues (5 mL/kg for acute respiratory distress syndrome [ARDS] to prevent barotraumas)
- *Inspiratory time (I-time):* 0.5 to 1 second (short I-time for asthmatics to allow maximum time for exhalation)
- *Peak pressures:* Keep under 40 cm H_2O (if >40 to 50, switch to pressure-controlled ventilation)
- *FIO_2:* Keep under 50% to 60%; if greater than 50% to 60%, then add PEEP (especially with ARDS)

8. What are the *normal* respiratory values and indications for mechanical ventilation?

- Vital capacity (mL/kg) = 65 to 75
- Maximum inspiratory pressure (MIP) to produce cough (cm H_2O) = −50 to −100
- Maximum expiratory pressure (MEP) for adequate cough (cm H_2O) = +100
- Tidal volume (mL/kg) = 5 to 8

- Respiratory rate (RR) (breaths/min) = 12 to 20
- Forced expired volume (FEV) in 1 second (mL/kg) = 50 to 60
- Minute ventilation (V_E = Respiratory rate × Tidal volume) = <10 L/min
- Peak expiratory flow rate (PEFR): 350 to 600 L/min

9. **What are the *abnormal and critical respiratory* values and indications for mechanical ventilation?**

- Vital capacity (mL/kg) = <15
- MIP = 0 to –20
- MEP = < +40
- V_t (mL/kg) = <5
- RR (breaths/min) = >35 or <8
- FEV in 1 second (mL/kg) = <10
- V_E (V_E = Respiratory rate × Tidal volume) = >10 L/min
- Unable to sustain normal Pa_{CO_2}.
- PEFR = 75 to 100 L/min (increased airway resistance, such as in an asthmatic attack)

10. **What are *normal* respiratory values when monitoring a ventilated patient?**

VENTILATION (Pa_{CO_2})
- pH = 7.35 to 7.45
- Pa_{CO_2} (mm Hg) = 35 to 45 (sea level)
- V_d/V_t (where V_d = dead space) = 0.3 to 0.4
- For example, if V_d/V_t = 0.6, then with a V_t of 1000 mL, only 40% is participating in gas exchange and 60% is not in contact with the pulmonary capillary bed; $\dot{V}/\dot{Q}$ mismatching may be seen with pulmonary emboli or injury

OXYGENATION (Pa_{O_2})
- Pa_{O_2} (mm Hg) = 80 to 100 (sea level)
- Alveolar-to-arterial oxygen difference on minimal O_2: 3 to 30
- $P(A–a)O_2$ (alveolar-arterial oxygen gradient) (mm Hg): 0.75
- Pa_{O_2}/Fi_{O_2} (Tobin index) = 475

11. **What are abnormal respiratory values when monitoring a ventilated patient?**

VENTILATION
- pH = <7.25
- Pa_{CO_2} (mm Hg) = >55 and rising
- V_d/V_t = >0.6 – increase in V_d

OXYGENATION (Pa_{O_2})
- Pa_{O_2} (mm Hg) = <70 (on O_2)
- Alveolar-to-arterial oxygen difference = >450 (on O_2)
- $P(A–a)O_2$ (mm Hg) = <0.15
- Pa_{O_2}/Fi_{O_2} (Tobin index) = <200

12. **What parameters are used to monitor the ventilator patient?**

- Oxygen (O_2) saturation: normal is greater than 90% and is used to evaluate for hypoxemia. These probes are only useful for saturations greater than 80%; if reading is less than this, an arterial blood gas (ABG) measurement should be obtained. Obtain ABG measurement 15 minutes after start of ventilation or any changes in settings.
- Goals during mechanical ventilation
  - Maintain pH between 7.35 and 7.45.
  - Maintain Pao_2 between 60 and 90 mm Hg.
  - Maintain $Paco_2$ between 25 and 45 mm Hg.
  - Normal minute ventilation (V_E)
  - Oxygen delivery

13. **What clinical conditions may lead to a low perfusion state?**

- Hypovolemia
- Hypothermia
- Peripheral vasoconstriction secondary to vasopressors
- Heart-lung bypass
- Intravenous (IV) dyes
- Nail polish and occasional dark-skinned subjects
- Dysfunctional hemoglobin

14. **How does the Sao_2 affect the Pao_2?**

According to the sigmoidal oxyhemoglobin dissociation curve for arterial blood, with greater than 90% saturation, the Pao_2 rises without much change in the Sao_2; below 80% saturation, the Pao_2 falls quickly.

15. **What is minute ventilation (V_E)?**

Minute ventilation is respiratory rate times tidal volume ($V_E = RR \times V_t$). V_E is increased in patients with lung disorders that lead to increased V_d. The normal V_E for men is 4 times the body surface area (BSA), and the normal V_E for women is 3.5 times the BSA.

16. **What controls oxygen delivery and $\dot{V}/\dot{Q}$ mismatch?**

Oxygen delivery and ventilation mismatch is controlled by the amount of oxygen and the mean airway pressure. By increasing the mean airway pressure, there is recruitment of alveoli.

17. **What is plateau pressure?**

Plateau pressure is a function of elastance alone. It is the pressure measurement at the end of inspiration when the ventilator is paused, which equals end-inspiratory pause. This inspiratory pause can be used to improve distribution of gas and oxygenation. Keep plateau pressure less than 50 cm H_2O or, in ARDS patients, less than 30 cm H_2O.

18. What is the I:E ratio?

The I:E ratio is time of inspiration (seconds) to time of expiration (seconds). Start at 1:2 to keep the effects of positive pressure reduced. Ratios of 1:1 or 1.7:1 improve PaO_2 without changing lung volumes in ARDS patients.

19. What is an inverse I:E ratio?

A 2:1 or 3:1 ratio is used to improve oxygenation in patients with ARDS.

20. What is static compliance?

Static compliance is the ease with which the lung distends. Compliance is defined as the change of volume that corresponds to the change in pressure. Normal compliance of the lungs is the sum of the compliance of both the lung tissue and surrounding thoracic structures such as the lungs, diaphragm, abdominal organs, and rib cage. The value of compliance varies depending on position, posture, and level of consciousness of a patient.

21. What are normal compliance values?

- Normal compliance values = 50 to 170 L/cm H_2O
- The values for intubated patients are as follows:
  - Males: 50 to 70 mL/cm H_2O to 100 mL/cm H_2O
  - Females: 35 to 45 mL/cm H_2O to 100 mL/cm H_2O

Static compliance in patients with chronic obstructive pulmonary disease (COPD) or asthma may have a higher threshold for what is considered to be decreased static compliance because their plateau pressures and V_ts are increased.

22. Describe the ventilator modes.

Ventilator Modes

Ventilator Modes	Weaning Modes	Mechanics/Uses	Advantages	Disadvantages
Assist control	No	Preset RR and V_t Triggered by patient's breath or set breath is given	Increased support. Safe minimum minute ventilation.	May lead to hyperventilation.* Keep sensitivity low to prevent triggering unnecessary breaths.

*Sedation may be used to prevent respiratory alkalosis.

Ventilator Modes—cont'd

Ventilator Modes	Weaning Modes	Mechanics/Uses	Advantages	Disadvantages
Pressure control	No	Breath controlled by pressure only	Pressure limited. Decreased risk of barotrauma and alveolar distention. Improves gas distribution and O_2 delivery.	Requires sedation. No guaranteed V_t.
Pressure-regulated volume control	No	Volume-controlled Assist control mode Deliver set flow rate to deliver a set volume at or below the maximum pressure	Guaranteed tidal volume, minimal barotrauma. Easily tolerated in awake patients.	None.
Spontaneous intermittent mechanical ventilation	Yes	Set breath delivered at a fixed interval; breaths in between not assisted	Variable amount of work of breathing may reduce alkalosis associated with assist control. Prevents muscle atrophy. Lowers peak airway pressures. Allows patient to gain strength.	Hypercapnia, fatigue, tachypnea with low rate. Increased work of breathing with spontaneous breaths unless pressure support is added.
Pressure support (continuous positive end-expiratory pressure ventilation [CPAP])	Yes	Provides constant pressure of gas once patient inspires	Overcomes resistance of endotracheal tube (ETT). Amount of pressure set depends on age, size of ETT, and size of chest wall.	Flow rate is high, which may be uncomfortable to patient.

23. What settings on the ventilator affect the cardiovascular system?

PEEP

Increased pressure in the lungs to support oxygenation is transmitted to intra-thoracic structures such as the vessels returning blood flow to the heart as well as the heart itself. This pressure can impede blood flow back to the heart and therefore the cardiac output decreases and is compromised. The PEEP affects the pressure on the heart more than positive-pressure ventilation alone. For example, assist control ventilation decreases cardiac output more than PEEP and IMV/SIMV/pressure support (continuous positive airway pressure [CPAP]) modes of ventilation.

I:E RATIO

If this ratio is reversed, the mean airway pressures are elevated in the lungs due to prolonged inspiratory times and decreased expiratory times. As a result, blood return to the heart is compromised and cardiac output decreases.

24. Describe the strategies used for mechanical ventilation.

Mechanical Ventilation	
Traditional	**Lung Protective**
V_t = 8 to 10 mL/kg	V_t = 5 to 8 mL/kg
Peak pressure <50 cm H_2O	Plateau pressure <35
Keep FiO_2 <60%	Hypercapnia allowed, pH 7.2 to 7.4
pH 7.36 to 7.44	

25. Describe how to troubleshoot the ventilator alarms.

- Determine reason for increased peak airway pressures.
  - Endotracheal tube obstruction or kink: check tube for obstructions or kinks.
  - Build up of secretions: suction for secretions.
  - Bronchospasm: give inhalers or bronchodilators.
- Determine cause of increased peak and plateau pressures.
  - Pneumothorax
  - Lobar atelectasis
  - Acute pulmonary edema
  - Worsening pneumonia
  - ARDS
  - COPD with tachypnea and auto-PEEP
  - Increased abdominal pressure
  - Asynchronous breathing
- Determine cause of decreased peak pressures.
  - System leak: check tubing for disconnection to patient.
  - Cuff leak: manually inflate cuff.
  - Hyperventilation

- Determine cause of increased V_E.
  - Presence of auto-PEEP
  - Poor $\dot{V}/\dot{Q}$ mismatching in the nonhomogenous lung
  - Changes in venous return
    Change to SIMV mode with presssure support (PS).
    Decrease PEEP.
    Change I:E ratio by increasing the expiratory phase of respiration.

26. What complications are associated with mechanical ventilation?

- Oxygen toxicity
- Decreased cardiac output
- Pneumonia and sepsis
- Psychological problems
- Ventilator dependence
- Oversedation and weaning difficulties
- Sinusitis
- Laryngeal damage
- Aspiration
- Tracheal necrosis
- Alveolar rupture: pneumothorax, pneumomediastinum, subcutaneous emphysema

27. How is respiratory alkalosis treated?

- Decrease both the ventilator rate and tidal volume as tolerated.
- If using assist control, change to SIMV.
- Change the trigger valve on the ventilator (for breaths) to be less sensitive.
- Administer sedation or pain medication (if due to increased RR from anxiety or pain).

28. What is ventilator-associated pneumonia?

Most commonly caused by aspiration, nosocomial pneumonias occur at a rate of 20% in intubated patients. Intubation alone introduces gram-negative bacteria into the airways. Poor suctioning techniques as well as a decreased cough or a circuit that has not been changed on a regular basis can predispose a patient to pneumonia. The fatality rate is as high as 43% to 70% in ventilated patients with pneumonia compared with 25% to 29% in ventilated patients without pneumonia.

29. How is ventilator-associated pneumonia treated?

Only treat the pneumonia if the patient has an elevated white blood cell count, fever, new infiltrates seen on chest radiograph, or change in character or amount of sputum production. Obtain culture to identify the organism responsible either from a tracheal aspirate or bronchial lavage.

30. What organisms are most commonly associated with ventilator-associated pneumonia?

- Gram-negative aerobes: *Pseudomonas, Klebsiella, Escherichia coli, Enterobacter, Serratia, Acinetobacter, Proteus mirabilis,* and *Haemophilus influenzae*
- Gram-positive aerobes: *Staphylococcus aureus, Streptococcus pneumoniae*
- Gram-negative anaerobes: *Bacteroides fragilis*
- Other: *Legionella pneumophila*
- Fungi: *Candida* species

31. What parameters are followed when weaning a patient from the ventilator?

- PaO_2/FIO_2: >400
- V_t: 5 to 7 mL/kg
- RR: 14 to 18 breaths/min or <25 breaths/min (head trauma is evaluated differently; RR may be high due to dysregulation in the central nervous system)
- V_E: 5 to 7 L/min or <10 L/min
- Vital capacity: 65 to 75 mL/kg or >10 mL/kg
- MIP: –20 to –30 cm H_2O

32. How is the Index of Rapid and Shallow Breathing RR/V_t used to predict weaning success?

- RR/V_t >105 = 95% wean attempts are unsuccessful
- RR/V_t <105 = 80% when attempts are successful

33. What complications may be associated with weaning from the ventilator?

- Dyspnea
- Anxiety
- Decreased cardiac output leading to pulmonary edema
- Electrolyte depletion
- Overfeeding
- Increased sedation
- Sepsis/pneumonia
- Acid-base imbalances
- Anemia
- Fluid balance
- Sleep deprivation

🔑 Key Points

- Positive pressure ventilation may be associated with barotrauma, resulting in pulmonary interstitial emphysema, pneumomediastinum, and tension pneumothorax.
- An exaggerated respiratory variation on the arterial pressure waveform is an indicator that positive pressure ventilation is affecting venous return and cardiac output.
- Clinical criteria for mechanical ventilation usually include apnea, respiratory distress with alteration in mentation, increased work of breathing, and obtundation with need for airway protection.

Internet Resources

EMedicine: Ventilator Management:
www.emedicine.com/emerg/topic788.htm

Rehab Info Network: Ventilation Management:
www.rehabinfo.net/resources/ventilation/management/management.asp

Acute Respiratory Distress Syndrome Support Center:
www.ards.org

Bibliography

Gupta, A. Mechanical ventilation: Things "I" wish I knew when I was an intern (n.d.). Retrieved November 10, 2003, from http://www.medslides.com/member/PulmonaryMedicine & Critical Care/Mech_Vent_AG.ppt.

Pilbeam, S.P. (1998). Establishing the need for mechanical ventilation. In J. Russell (Ed.), *Mechanical Ventilation: Physiological and clinical applications* (pp. 175-223). St. Louis: Mosby.

Tegtmeyer, K. (1998). Initial mechanical ventilation. Retrieved November 1, 2003, from http://www.peds.umn.edu/divisions/pccm/teaching/acp/vents.html.

Chapter 22

End-of-Life Issues

Megan E. Carr

1. What are the nuances of legal terminology when patients are no longer autonomous?

To better understand the complex nature of end-of-life care, it is important to have clarity in the common terminology defining the most crucial aspects that may direct patient care.

POWER OF ATTORNEY

Power of attorney is a right that is given by one competent individual to another, granting that person the right to do a specific act for the competent individual, such as write checks, open bank accounts, or sign legal documents. A power of attorney ceases to be in effect if the competent individual revokes the power of attorney or becomes incapacitated, unless that person has executed a durable power of attorney (Romano, 1998).

DURABLE POWER OF ATTORNEY

A durable power of attorney is a specific document in which a competent individual, before his or her incapacitation, names another person to act on his or her behalf once that individual is unable to manage his or her own affairs. The person designated as durable power of attorney also has the role of serving as guardian of the individual without the necessity of petitioning the court to have the individual declared incapacitated in the event of a medical disability.

GUARDIANSHIP

Guardianship is a legal relationship between one individual (the guardian) and the incapacitated individual (the ward) that gives the guardian the right and the duty to act on behalf of the incapacitated party in making decisions that affect that person's life. Unless the terms of guardianship are limited by the court in some way, the guardian manages all of the incapacitated party's personal, legal, and financial affairs.

INCAPACITATED PERSON

An incapacitated person is an adult whose "ability to receive and evaluate information effectively and communicate decisions in any way is impaired to such a significant extent that he is partially or totally unable to manage his financial resources or meet essential requirements for his physical health and safety" (Romano, 1998). The determination of incapacitation, then, is made by a court-appointed judge who reviews supportive documentation provided by the treating clinician. There is no specific need to have this documentation provided by a psychiatrist. The court will accept a report or testimony that a clinician who has examined the patient can give an opinion, based upon medical certainty, as to whether or not a guardian is necessary.

2. What is a living will and how can it be executed?

A living will is a document that sets forth important definitions in the limits of care a person deems appropriate for himself. By virtue of drafting a living will, an individual truly may direct his or her own care considering, of course, that the person has shared this document with their designated surrogate. Typically defined terms in a living will include the following: incompetence, terminal condition, permanently unconscious, life-sustaining treatment, revocation, and designation of attending physician or health care provider (Romano, 1998). Interestingly, revocation, by which the individual retracts previously made statements, can be made "without regard to the declarant's (current) mental or physical condition."

Execution of a living will may be made by any individual of sound mind who is 18 years of age or older, or who has graduated from high school or is married. This declaration must be voluntarily executed by the individual or other authorized person and must be witnessed by two individuals who are at least 18 years of age.

A living will only becomes effective when a copy of the declaration is provided to the person's attending physician or health care institution.

3. What is informed consent and how may it relate to surrogate decision makers?

Central to the concept of patient autonomy is the requirement that the patient be capable of making medical decisions. Combined with this notion is the well-established legal principle that health care practitioners, including paramedics and emergency medical technicians, are responsible for making adequate disclosure of information to the patient and obtain informed consent.

Included in disclosure, the health care professional must discuss the following:
· Diagnosis, nature and purpose of treatment
· Desired outcome
· Hazards or risk of the medication
· Treatment or proposed health care
· Chances of success or failure
· Alternative procedures that could achieve the desired medical result
· Likely medical consequences of no treatment (Romano, 1998)

When a patient is deemed "incompetent," surrogate decision makers may be placed in a situation to confer consent. The same general principles apply for clinicians to obtain consent from surrogates as apply for clinicians to obtain primary patient consent. If a living will exists, clinicians and surrogates are obligated to follow the patient's directive. In emergency situations, implied consent is activated until such time as a surrogate or the patient is able to communicate wishes for pursuing future care.

4. What are the medical obligations of acute care practitioners?

Clinicians make a commitment to each patient that has as its foremost objective two principles: (1) beneficence (being of benefit to the patient), and (2) non-maleficence (doing no harm). The scope of responsibilities of health care providers that comes as a result of those two principles are as follows:
- To promote health and well-being by preventing and curing disease
- To alleviate pain and suffering
- To do so in ways that are caring and respectful of the patient's dignity and worth as a human being by respecting his or her right to self-determination

Although the respect for patient autonomy is forefront in a clinician's care with regard to limiting care by refusing treatment, antithetically it does not entitle patients, or families for that matter, to *demand* inappropriately aggressive care. Whereas the limitation of providing medically futile care has been supported by professional organizations representing intensive care unit (ICU) clinicians, others have challenged it because of the inconsistently applied terms defining *futility*.

One position is that the purpose of life-sustaining therapy should be to restore or sustain *meaningful* survival, where meaningful refers to a survival that the patient can appreciate and value (DeLisser & Lanken, 2001).

The following figure depicts decision making for the patient who cannot speak for himself or herself.

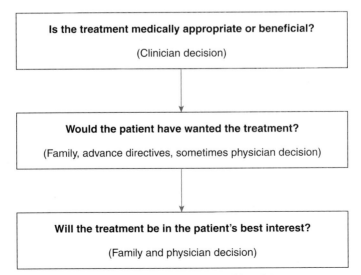

Decision making for patients unable to participate in care.

5. **What are the legal and ethical ramifications of the Right-to-Die Amendment for acute care practitioners?**

Passed by the federal government in December 1991, the Patient Self-Determination Act, (commonly referred to as the Right-to-Die Amendment) requires health care facilities to advise newly admitted patients of their right to refuse or accept treatment if they become gravely ill. This act applies to most health care providers including hospitals, skilled nursing facilities, home health agencies, hospices, and prepaid organizations that accept Medicaid or Medicare (Romano, 1998). While the Patient Self-Determination Act does not require a competency determination, a health care provider would be prudent to first determine the issue of competency before discussing authority to treat, living wills, or health care directives.

6. **Define euthanasia versus palliative terminal care.**

Euthanasia has typically been defined as active measures to hasten death in an attempt to alleviate suffering of a chronic or terminal illness. Alternatively, palliative care addresses the need to aggressively manage symptoms associated with a terminal condition without actively pursuing measures that would result in premature death. The gray zone between the two definitions occurs when the treatment of symptoms, with such things as opiates, may hasten the dying process while treating a frightening symptom, such as dyspnea.

Awareness of the inadequacies of the care that is provided at the end-of-life makes it not surprising to find that if people are asked "Are you in favor of euthanasia?" a majority reply that they are. Further questioning may reveal, however, that they would rather die painlessly (Hendin, 2002).

When a knowledgeable clinician addresses the desperation and suffering that underlie the request for assisted suicide and assures the patient that he or she will continue to do so until the end, most patients change their minds (Kaplan, Snyder & Faber-Langendoen, 2000).

Currently, euthanasia is not a legal option in the United States. Ironically, opposition to legalization in the United States is strongest among clinicians who know the most about caring for terminally ill patients (oncologists, gerontologists, and palliative care clinicians, including nurse practitioners). In varying degrees, compassion for suffering patients and respect for patient autonomy serve as the basis for the strongest arguments in favor of legalization. Compassion, however, does not guarantee against doing no harm.

7. **How can clinicians provide more culturally sensitive end-of-life care?**

Practicing health care in the United States offers the unique challenge of caring for patients from a multitude of ethnic backgrounds. These differences in beliefs, values, and traditional health care practices are of particular relevance at the end-of-life. To provide the comprehensive care that is so critical at the end-of-life, it is imperative that clinicians use resources to address these multifaceted issues (Crawley et al., 2002).

Effective strategies include the following:
- Addressing a language barrier, if there is one, and having a medical interpreter available to ensure thorough explanation of medical issues and to maximize communication efforts
- Acknowledging the patient's heritage by allowing cultural symbols (including music) to be displayed or used in the patient's room
- Including the family in discussions regarding care (often the family can even bring in ethnic food that is not necessarily available in the hospital and would provide much needed nutrition)
- Allowing family members to stay overnight in the patient's room, in particular when death is imminent

When strategizing a comprehensive plan of care for a patient of any ethnicity, it is reassuring to know that "For every road there is a map that exists or can be made" (Personal communication, J. Reifsnyder, May 12, 1995).

8. How can clinicians effectively integrate the religious preferences of patients in end-of life care?

Clinicians are astute medical history gatherers. Unfortunately, a key component of a person's history, their religious preference, is often overlooked when they are admitted to the acute care setting. Some patients are more open in sharing their religious preferences than others, but an astute clinician can tune into subtle, or sometimes not so subtle clues about their religious background. This may have significant implications for their future medical care, particularly end-of-life care, in that religious preferences often dictate how a person chooses to assimilate the care plan that has been designed for them.

In the 1995 SUPPORT (Study to Understand Prognoses and Preferences for Outcomes and Risks of Treatment) trial, there was a consensus statement that identified the assessment and support of spiritual and religious well-being and management of spiritual and religious problems as core principles of professional practice and care at the end-of-life (Daaleman & VandeCreek, 2000).

As challenging as it is sometimes to incorporate the religious value set of a patient in an acute care setting, particularly in intensive care, it is prudent to do so. In end-of-life care, religion and religious traditions serve two primary functions: the provision of a set of core beliefs about life events and the establishment of an ethical foundation for clinical decision making (Stotland, 1999). In many irreversible medical situations, it may be the only intervention a clinician may be able to offer.

9. How do the major religions view death?

To summarize the leading religious views on death, the following information may be useful for clinicians (Sloan & Bagiella, 1999):

BUDDHISM

From its inception, Buddhism has stressed the importance of death, because awareness of death is what prompted the Buddha to perceive the ultimate futility of worldly concerns and pleasures. While dying, the person can be surrounded by friends, family, and monks who can recite Buddhists scriptures and mantras to help the person achieve a peaceful state of mind.

CHRISTIANITY

For Christians whose lives are guided by the Bible, the reality of death is acknowledged as part of the human condition, affected by sin. While waiting for death, family and friends are very much welcome and often celebrate in the passing of life in the hopes of eternal salvation.

HINDUISM

Followers believe in the rebirth and reincarnation of souls. Therefore, death is not seen as an end, but as a natural process in the existence of souls that will continue after the current soul has been placed to rest. Rituals that are important for clinicians to be sensitive to include the final bath. It may be important for the family to supervise this act, or even help with the final preparation of the body to the morgue.

ISLAM

When death approaches, the close family and friends try to support and comfort the dying person through supplication as well as remembrance of Allah and the will of Allah. The attendance is to help the dying person iterate his commitment to the unity of God.

JUDAISM

Believers of Judaism have stressed the natural fact of death and its role in giving life meaning. The fear of death, concern about the fate of one's own soul and those of loved ones, and ethical concerns that some people die unfairly, have been well described in the Jewish literature. For Orthodox believers, it is important for the family and Rabbi to be present when a person dies and to actively participate or supervise the preparation of the body.

10. What are the economic implications for providing more aggressive care in the acute care and critical care settings?

It is estimated that end-of-life care consumes 10% to 12% of all health care expenditures and 27% of Medicare expenditures (Iglehart, 1999). Furthermore, the number of Medicare enrollees is expected to grow considerably in the next 20 years, raising considerable concerns over the anticipated costs of providing care to an increasingly older adult population.

As the national debate about health care costs, access, and quality continues, there is an increasing need to turn to economic analysis for assistance in deciding resource allocation, particularly with regard to end-of-life care. Decisions regarding the delivery of health care at the end-of-life underscore the inherent conflict between economics and bioethics. In fact, there has been much controversy and confusion about how much money, if any, can be saved by the implementation of advance directives and hospice programs. A widely quoted article showed that Medicare patients with advance directives had a 68% reduction in mean hospital charges for their terminal hospitalizations. Additionally, it was found by the National Hospice Study that there was an average savings of $0.68 for every dollar spent among those who used hospice in the last month of life (Emanuel, 1996).

With this information in mind, rationing itself is not denounced as ethically unacceptable, so long as the deprivation of services provided is egalitarian. This attitude contrasts with British National Health Services guidelines that explicitly refuse specific health care services to patients because of advanced age or illness (Pronovost & Angus, 2001).

As advancements in technology continue, there are more and more machines to offer patients. Clinicians are in the unique position of having to decide when it is efficacious and ethical to offer such options to patients. The mere cost is not often considered in the decision, but the equitable use of the treatment option must be considered strongly before initiation.

11. What are some societal concerns regarding fairness and resource allocation?

Associated with the economic implications of using health care resources, clinicians must also be sensitive to the fair allocation of health care resources. Decisions to allocate scarce resources can be ethical and appropriate if they involve the application of institution-wide criteria supported by a societal consensus, such as those rules applied when organs are transplanted. However, the current system of U.S. medical care has no universally accepted criteria for allocation of hospital resources. Therefore the limits of care that one clinician imposes on his or her patients may not be necessarily shared by other clinicians or patients in similar situations. As a result, health care providers have an obligation to know the costs of interventions that they use and use them wisely and to advocate for fair and equal access to ICU and other essential health care resources for those in need.

12. When is it appropriate to approach the subject of organ donation with the family of a terminally ill patient?

Anyone who has cared for critically ill patients has, perhaps often, encountered a situation in which a patient has suffered irreversible brain damage that rendered that patient "brain dead." Considering the comprehensive health history of the individual, it may be appropriate to consider organ donation.

Because it is often a sudden event that results in the terminal condition of the individual, broaching the subject of donation is often a difficult discussion to have. Sometimes families who are approached too soon consider the medical team is "giving up" on their loved one and only are considering the option of harvesting organs. It is therefore crucial to use the resources available in organ procurement organizations to assist with the concept of donation if that is indeed a viable option. Skilled practitioners who are expert at discussing the organ donation process as well as grief counseling are available for this particular purpose.

There are situations in which a patient has formally designated his or her wishes to donate organs by virtue of signing a formal organ donor card or designation of such on a driver's license, and the family decides to override the designation and not to donate their loved ones organs. Under current organ procurement allocation rules in the United States, in this instance, the family's decision would only trump the previously determined decision if there were no witnesses to authorize donation. It is therefore imperative to share the decision to donate with family members or significant others who may have to make the ultimate decision to donate (Stacey Doll, Gift of Life Hospital Liaison, Personal Communication, December 23, 2003).

13. How can the acute care nurse practitioner foster better patient and family communication?

The acute care and intensive care unit settings represent a hospital setting in which death and discussion about end-of-life care are common, yet these conversations are often difficult. In fact, it has been estimated that, of patients who die in the hospital, approximately half are cared for in an ICU within 3 days of their death and one third spend greater than 10 days in the ICU during their final hospitalization. In this setting, many studies have demonstrated that the majority of deaths in the ICU involve withholding or withdrawing multiple life-sustaining therapies (Curtis et al., 2001).

In the 1980s and 1990s, clinicians and legislators alike believed that advance directives would serve as a means of communication of the level of care patients wished from their clinicians (Curtis et al., 2001). If completed successfully, these directives would theoretically obviate the need for acute care clinicians to discuss end-of-life care with patients and families because their wishes would already have been conveyed. This has not been the case.

Prior studies have shown that less than 5% of ICU patients are able to communicate with clinicians at the time that decisions are made about withholding or withdrawing life-sustaining therapies (Edmonds & Rogers, 2003). Therefore when ICU clinicians must discuss these issues, they often discuss them with patients' families or surrogate decision makers. It often is the responsibility of the bedside nurse or the acute care nurse practitioner to facilitate such a discussion that involves the multidisciplinary team including specialists (e.g., cardiology, neurology), therapists, social workers, and sometimes the ethics committee.

Evaluation measures of clinician conversation about end-of-life discussions have identified substantial shortcomings. Content discussed, including patient's diagnosis, prognosis, or treatment options, were estimated as being poorly understood at the completion of a meeting. Additionally, it has been noted that clinicians spend an average of 75% of the time talking and missed important opportunities to discuss personal values and goals of therapy (Heyland et al., 2003).

To facilitate an effective meeting, therefore, it is encouraged that the environment be supportive to foster listening. If possible, including the patient in the discussion should be a priority. Therefore, even simple tasks such as waiting for a procedure to be completed to allow for patient modesty, arranging chairs in the room to make it more conducive for a comfortable discussion arena, turning off pagers, and maybe even having pastoral care available can create the supportive environment that will allow family members and patients alike to actively listen and participate in such a discussion that is focused on the patient goals and to honor the patient's wishes and dignity.

Just as important as the first meeting is that of continued discussions that allow for updates and modifications of the plan of care, in particular with regard to comfort care measures. If patients and families have been provided the information they need to make informed decisions, they are more able to adjust the plan if the clinical situation changes for the worse.

14. What are the limitations and obligations of a Do Not Resuscitate order?

Since the enactment of the Patient Self-Determination Act in 1990, advance directives have become a part of clinical practice in critical care units. Even though many people say that they have discussed health care choices with family members and friends, interestingly, only approximately 2% to 15% of adults in the United States have a formal advance directive that has been officially drafted and witnessed by key members who can effectively use the document (Ott, 1999).

Limitations that have been discovered with regard to drafting the actual document include clinician beliefs that advance directives are unnecessary for young, "healthy" patients and clinician lack of knowledge about how to formulate advance directives. Because it is often the primary care clinician who initiates such conversations, time constraints with HMO-driven practices have also been described as limitations to effective designation.

When patients have not made their decisions well known or even made the fact that they have an advance directive known to likely parties who may ultimately have to make end-of-life decisions for them, the truest intent of an advance directive is lost. In some instances, the proxy decision maker may not be the family, which may cause much controversy at the bedside when crucial choices need to be made.

The more practical limitation to an effective advance directive is that oftentimes the generic versions that are available through most hospital admission processes or stationary stores do not delineate specific wishes for care. Because no one can ever predict the manner in which every possible clinical scenario will pan out, there is going to be room for interpretation with any directive a person could make.

15. **When is it appropriate to transition care to or enlist the services of a palliative care team in the acute care setting?**

With cure as the goal for so many patients to enter the acute care setting in the first place, sometimes it is difficult for both patients and clinicians alike to acknowledge when that is no longer possible to achieve.

Palliative care teams developed from the need to achieve better symptom management for patients who may have been referred to hospice care too late to derive significant symptom management (Emanuel, 1996). Services provided by palliative care teams incorporate all aspects of comfort including the following: depression and anxiety, intractable nausea and vomiting, maximizing pain management while attempting not to oversedate, and oftentimes, dyspnea management.

Comprising the palliative care team are often anesthesiologists, pain management nurse practitioners, former hospice nurses, pharmacists, social workers, and even massage therapists. Even though the bedside nurse and other clinicians can provide many of these services, this team offers a plethora of additional options that may be tailored to one specific patient's symptom management needs and be exactly what makes an appropriate transition from aggressive care to end-of-life care. This is especially true if the goal of going home is no longer an option.

16. **Should health care teams include families and support persons in terminal resuscitative events?**

This topic has been a source of much controversy. Even though it is somewhat disturbing to envision a loved one being actively resuscitated, it may be what some families need to provide closure and feel assured that all measures were employed to attempt to save their loved one if aggressive measures were being pursued, or if palliation is the goal, that the respects of the individual patient were honored.

Alternatively, it is concerning to clinicians that this strategy may allow for litigation or seemingly interfere with resuscitation because the family "gets in the way."

Interestingly, a recent study indicates that patients who had family members present at the time of death also were more likely to have DNR orders written, to have treatments, such as mechanical ventilation, withdrawn, and to receive narcotics before death (Tschann, Kaufman, & Micco, 2003).

17. **How can the acute care health care team collaborate with hospice to facilitate more aggressive inpatient palliative care?**

Although the numbers of patients who die while being cared for by a hospice have been rising slowly, patients do not generally spend enough time in these programs to experience all the potential benefits. In fact, in 1995, although the median length of stay was 36 days, nearly one fifth of patients died within a week of admission (Emanuel, 1996).

Measures to facilitate in-patient hospice have been enlisted to maximize the true palliative goal of hospice and to hopefully erase the stigma that seems to be associated with "hospice". The criteria of life expectancy have been extended well beyond the traditional 6 months that used to define hospice according to Medicare. Therefore, clinicians in the acute care setting may be the ones to refer to hospice.

Depending on the patient and family's wishes, this care may be provided in the hospital setting first with the goal to transition to the home. Some families, however, may not be able to care for their loved one at home depending on the technical complexity of doing so. In this instance, purely using the in-patient hospice benefit is the best option. This allows for the caregivers to have the direct care needs met and have the immeasurable benefit of bereavement counseling offered for up to 1 year after their loved one dies (Personal Communication, Eve Brahman, Director Wisahickon Hospice, December 19, 2003).

18. **What is the role of the ethics committee in helping families discern differences among health care providers?**

Consultants are often brought in to offer opinions regarding their specialty as it relates to the patient's comprehensive care. Likewise, there are difficult situations that arise when patients, or more commonly their families, demand ICU interventions that the patient's attending physician and other members of the team do not believe would be beneficial or otherwise indicated.

When agreement with a surrogate decision maker still cannot be reached despite following appropriate steps of communication that have been described previously, it may be appropriate to involve the ethics committee to apply the futility standard, if the institution's policy permits (see the figure on p. 270). This relieves the primary clinician of unilateral decision making and allows for an objective opinion to be interjected for both parties. In some instances, it may offer the family the opportunity to transfer the patient's care to another clinician who is willing to provide the disputed intervention.

With the variety of consultants able to "weigh in" on a given clinical situation, it is often confusing for the family to know which opinion is appropriate to consider "gospel" and therefore the appropriate way in which to proceed. Oftentimes there may also be an element of unresolved and unappreciated feelings of guilt, anger, fear, or denial, particularly of family members who

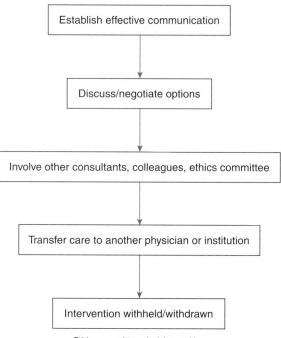

Establish effective communication

Discuss/negotiate options

Involve other consultants, colleagues, ethics committee

Transfer care to another physician or institution

Intervention withheld/withdrawn

Ethics committee: decision making.

have been estranged from the patient before the ICU admission that drives the decision to press forward with all possible interventions (appropriate or not). To include a nonpartisan assessment by an ethics committee as part of comprehensive plan of care may often allow for successful resolution of a seemingly irreconcilable situation.

19. What is the role of debriefing in managing end-of-life issues?

Because acute care nurse practitioners are primarily used to directing care toward saving lives, it is often a sense of frustration or even failure that patient care shift from cure to comfort. The daily demands on clinicians are physically and emotionally exhausting at times. Whereas several studies have been performed to address the patient and family needs at the end-of-life, there are few that address the needs of nurses who care for this challenging population (Kirchhoff et al., 2000).

It has been described that the most efficacious way in which to deal with the stresses of intensive care includes debriefing sessions (Day, 2001). Scenarios that were best used included a multidisciplinary approach to care in which each team member was able to discuss his or her respective vantage point. Physician colleagues, respiratory, physical and occupational therapists, and bedside nurses all have a hand in implementing patient care and all should be included in a debriefing session if possible immediately following a patient death, particularly an unexpected one. Additional resources of pastoral care and in some instances a psychiatric liaison have been noted to be instrumental in allowing clinicians to recognize their feelings with regard to a patient's death.

20. What is the Five Wishes approach toward living wills?

With recent court cases highlighting the shortcomings of generic advance directives, the need arose to develop a more specific version of a living will that would address the multitude of issues that are key to directing patient care and honoring patients' lives as human beings. Five Wishes was designed to meet that need and, in fact, is the first living will that specifically identifies personal, emotional, and spiritual needs as well as the direct issues of patient medical care.

Included in the design of the Five Wishes living will are detailed options for all aspects of end-of-life care. The wishes are delineated as follows:
- *Wish 1:* The Person I Want to Make Health Care Decisions for Me When I Can't Make Them for Myself.
- *Wish 2:* My Wish for the Kind of Medical Treatment I Want or Don't Want. Specifically addressed are the differences between life support, withdrawal of care, and permanent and irrecoverable brain injury or coma
- *Wish 3:* My Wish for How Comfortable I Want to Be
- *Wish 4:* My Wish for How I Want People to Treat Me
- *Wish 5:* My Wish for What I Want My Loved Ones to Know. This section also addresses the ways in which a person would like to be remembered as by a memorial service and identifies wishes to donate organs.

21. Is there a stepwise fashion by which clinicians can approach the withholding and withdrawal of life support?

Keeping some of the aforementioned tenets in mind, there is a comprehensive way in which to approach the difficult decision of withholding or withdrawing aggressive or even basic health care (DeLisser and Lanken, 2001):
- Determine if the patient had adequate decision-making capacity.
- Establish effective communication.
- Formulate the health care team's recommendation.
- Present the recommendations to the patient or family.
- Attempt to resolve conflicts.
- If conflicts cannot be resolved, consider applying the futility standard, if applicable and available.
- Withhold or withdraw life support with close attention to patient comfort and family needs.

22. What resources are available for clinicians to provide to patients, families and support persons faced with end-of-life care decisions?

Typically there are in-hospital educational resources that are available to both staff and laypersons, including library and Internet resources. This chapter includes a comprehensive list of websites that can further guide clinicians in giving end-of-life care. Clinicians who are expert in dealing with end-of-life issues include hospice liaisons, palliative care team members, clergy, and hospital ethics committee members. When questions or concerns arise outside your scope of practice or comfort level, never hesitate to use these valuable resources.

 Key Points

- The role of the acute care nurse practitioner is crucial in fostering an environment in which patients and caregivers can make difficult end-of-life decisions.
- Thorough and comprehensive communication between the clinical staff and patient and family is key in defining appropriate levels of care.
- Honoring the patient's autonomy, dignity, and wishes as an individual is the distinct privilege and challenge of the acute care nurse practitioner.
- While much has been accomplished with regard to improving end-of-life care, much more effort and research is needed to maximize this aspect of acute care.

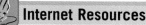 **Internet Resources**

Aging with Dignity (The Five Wishes Project):
www.agingwithdignity.org

American Academy of Hospice and Palliative Medicine:
www.aahpm.org

American College of Physicians: End-of-Life Care Consensus Project:
www.acponline.org/ethics/eolc.htm

American Colleges of Nursing: End-of-Life Care:
www.aacn.nche.edu/elnec

End of Life/Palliative Education Resource:
www.eperc.mcw.edu

Hospice and Palliative Nurses Association:
www.hpna.org

The Hospice of the Florida Suncoast:
www.thehospice.org

Hospice Foundation of America:
www.hospicefoundation.org

Internet Resources—cont'd

IIPCA- Initiative to Improve Palliative Care for African Americans:
www.soros.org/initiating/pdia/focus_areas/palliative_african

Innovations in End-of-Life Care:
www.edc.org/lastacts

Life's End Institute: Missoula Demonstration Project:
www.missoulademonstration.org

Center for Practical Bioethics:
www.midbio.org

National Hospice and Palliative Care Organization:
www.nhpco.org

National Resource Center on Diversity in End-of-Life Care:
www.nrcd.com

Partnership for Caring:
www.partnershipforcaring.org

Project on Death in America:
www.soros.org/initiatives/pdia

Promoting Excellence in End-of-Life Care:
www.promotingexcellence.org

Supportive Care of the Dying:
www.careofdying.org

The Washington Home Center for Palliative Care Studies:
www.medicaring.org

Working Group to Improve Psychosocial Care Near the End of Life:
www3.uakron.edu/eol

Zen Hospice Project:
www.zenhospice.org

Bibliography

Crawley, L.M., et al. (2002). Strategies for culturally effective end-of-life care. *Annals of Internal Medicine, 136*(9), 673-679.

Curtis, J., et al. (2001). The family conference as a focus to improve communication about end-of-life care in the intensive care unit: Opportunities for improvement. *Critical Care Medicine,* (29)2, 26-33.

Day, L. (2001). How nurses shift from care of a brain-injured patient to maintenance of a brain-dead organ donor. *American Journal of Critical Care,* (10)5, 306-312.

Daaleman, T., & VandeCreek, L. (2000). Placing religion and spirituality in end-of-life care. *JAMA, 284*(19), 2514-2517.

DeLisser, H., & Lanken, P. (2001). End-of-life care. In P.N. Lanken (Ed.), *The intensive care unit manual* (pp. 255-265). Philadelphia: W.B. Saunders.

Edmonds, P., & Rogers, A. (2003). "If only someone had told me…" A review of the care of patients dying in the hospital. *Clinical Medicine 3*(2), 149-152.

Emanuel, E. (1996). Cost savings at the end of life: What do the data show? *JAMA, 275*(24), 1907-1914.

Hendin, H. (2002). Assisted suicide, euthanasia, and the right to end-of-life care. *The Journal of Crisis Intervention and Suicide Prevention, 23*(1), 40-44.

Heyland, D., et al. (2003). Dying in the ICU: Perspectives of family members. *Chest, 124*(1), 392-397.

Iglehart, J.K. (1999). The American healthcare system: Medicare. *New England Journal of Medicine, 340*, 327-332.

Kaplan, A., Snyder, L., & Faber-Langendoen, K. (2000). The role of guidelines in the practice of physician assisted suicide. *Annals of Internal Medicine, 132*(6), 476-481.

Kirchhoff, K., et al. (2000). Intensive care nurses' experiences with end-of-life care. *American Journal of Critical Care, 9*(1), 36-42.

Ott, B. (1999). Advance directives: The emerging body of research. *American Journal of Critical Care, 8*(1), 514-519.

Pronovost, P., & Angus, D. (2001). Economics of end-of-life care in the intensive care unit. *Critical Care Medicine, 29*(2), N49-N51.

Romano, J. (1998). *Legal rights of the catastrophically ill and injured: A family guide* (2nd ed., pp. 10-46). Norristown, PA: Joseph L. Romano, Esquire.

Sloan, R.P., & Bagiella, E. (1999). Religion, spirituality and medicine. *The Lancet, 353*(9163), 664-667.

Stotland, N. (1999). When religion collides with medicine. *The American Journal of Psychiatry, 156*(2), 304-307.

SUPPORT Principal Investigators. (1995). A controlled trial to improve care for seriously ill hospitalized patients: The Study to Understand Prognoses and Preferences for Outcomes and Risks of Treatment (SUPPORT). *JAMA, 274*, 1591-1598.

Tschann, J.M., Kaufman, S.R., & Micco, G.P. (2003). Family involvement in end-of-life hospital care. *Journal of the American Geriatric Society, 51*(6), 835-840.

Index

A

Abdomen in chest radiograph, 45
Abdominal pain, 105
ABI, 27–28
Abiomed BVSW 5000I, 200, 201f
Absolute neutrophil count, 7
ACC/AHA guidelines, 27
Accessory muscles of respiration, 73
Acid-base disorder, 127, 127t
ACORN/CORCAP device, 93
Acute leukemia, 145–146
Acute pain, 233
Acute pyelonephritis, 126–127
Acute renal failure, 128, 129t
Acute stroke, 119
Addiction, 243
Adenosine in stress testing, 35
Adjuvant agent for pain, 237
Adrenal disorder, 67–68
Advanced cardiac support device, 199–213
Adverse effects of diabetes drug, 61t–62t
Agency for Healthcare Research and Quality, 97
Agitation, 223–225
Air bronchography, 46
Airway in chest radiograph, 44
Airway obstruction, reversible, 42
Alanine aminotransferase, 6
Alarm, ventilator, 254–255
Alcohol withdrawal syndrome, 230
Alkaline phosphatase, 6
Allergen, 219
Alpha-glucosidase inhibitor, 61, 62t
Alternative pain management, 243
Alveolar infiltrate, 46
American Cancer Society, 158–159
American College of Cardiology, 27, 28
American Heart Association, 27, 28, 158
Aminophylline, 220

Analgesia
    opioid, 225, 238–241
    patient-controlled, 238–239
Analgesic receptor, 235, 235t
Anaphylactic shock, 219–220
Anastomotic leak, 107
Anemia, 143, 145
    iron-deficiency, 7, 143t
    reticulocyte count in, 7
    types of, 143t–144t
Aneurysm
    aortic, 90–91
    cerebral, 116
Angina pectoris, 19–20, 34
Angiography
    for bleeding, 109
    in pulmonary embolus, 16
Angiotensin-converting enzyme inhibitor, 94
Anion gap, 5
Ankle-brachial blood pressure index, 27–28
Anteroposterior chest radiograph, 43
Antibiotic
    to prevent pneumonia, 74–75
    in skull fracture, 180
Anticoagulation
    in heparin-induced thrombocytopenia, 151
    with ventricular assist device, 209–210
Antidiuretic hormone
    diabetes insipidus and, 68–69
    inappropriate secretion of, 5
Antigen
    carcinoembryonic, 9
    human leukocyte, 8
    prostate-specific, 9, 158
Antihistamine for anaphylactic shock, 220
Anxiety, 223–225
Aorta in chest radiograph, 44
Aortic aneurysm, 90–91
Aortic dissection, 90–91

f indicate illustrations, and *t* indicates tabular material

Aortic dissection—*cont'd*
  magnetic resonance imaging in, 15
Aortic injury, 180–181
Aortic stenosis, 89–90
Aortoiliac disease, 139
Aplastic anemia, 144t
Arrhythmia
  postoperative, 95
  ventricular assist device and, 209
Arterial blood gases, 50–51
  in pulmonary embolus, 80
Arterial insufficiency, 140
Arterial stenosis, renal, magnetic resonance
  angiography of, 14
Arterial versus venous injury, 182–183
Artery disease, coronary. *See* Coronary artery
  disease
Arthritis
  osteoarthritis, 134
  rheumatoid, 133–134
Aspartate aminotransferase, 6
Aspiration, tube feeding and, 173, 174
Assessment
  nutritional, 169
  pain, 236
Asthma, 85–86
Atrial fibrillation, postoperative, 93, 95
Atrial myxoma, 93
Atorvastatin, 99
Atypical angina pectoris, 19–20
Atypical pneumonia, 75
Automatic mode ventricular assist device, 202
Autonomy, 261
Axis in electrocardiography, 23–24
Axonal injury, diffuse, 188t

B

B-type natriuretic peptide, 22
Bacillus
  gram-negative, 52–53
  gram-positive, 52
Bacteria, gram-negative and gram-positive,
  52–53
Balloon pump, intraaortic, 218
Bariatric surgery, 107
Barium swallow, video, 13
Basilar skull fracture, 180
Batwing pattern on chest radiograph, 47
Beck's triad, 181
Benzodiazepine
  for alcohol withdrawal syndrome, 230
  for anxiety, 225
Beraprost, 83

Beta-blocker
  for aortic aneurysm, 91
  for atrial fibrillation, 95
Bicuspid aortic valve, 89
Biguanide, 61
Bile duct scan, 13–14
Biliary colic, 106
Biopsy, cardiac, 36–37, 37t
Bleeding
  gastrointestinal, 15, 108–110
  intracranial, 118
Blood
  cardiac markers in, 28–29
  occult, 159
  in urethral meatus, 182
  in urine, 125
Blood disorder, 143–152
Blood gases, 50–51
  in pulmonary embolus, 80
Blood pressure, high, 100–101, 100t, 101t
  aortic dissection and, 91
  intra-abdominal hypertension and, 184
Blood test
  in coronary artery disease, 20
  liver function and, 6
Blown pupil, 179
Blue bloater, 76
Blunt trauma
  aortic, 180–181
  cardiac, 181
  pneumothorax and, 85
BMI, 169–170
Body mass index, 169–170, 170t
Bone loss, 156–157
Bosentan, 82–83
Bowel
  obstruction of, 107, 111t–112t
  penetrating trauma to, 189
Brain tumor, 119–120
Breakthrough pain, 237
Breast cancer
  prevention of, 157
  screening for, 158
Bronchitis, 75–77
Bronchography, air, 46
Brudzinski sign, 121
Buddhism, 263–264
BUN/creatinine ratio, 10
Bypass graft, coronary artery, 96–97

C

C-reactive protein, 22
CA 27.29 antigen, 9

Calcium
  cardiac, 13
  corrected, 7
  daily requirement of, 135t
  in osteoporosis, 135
Calculation of anion gap, 5
Cancer antigen, 9
Cancer pain, 238
Cancer screening, 158–160
Cannula for ventricular assist device, 205, 207
Carbon monoxide, 39
Carcinoembryonic antigen, 9
Cardiac biopsy grading system, 37t
Cardiac calcium scoring, 13
Cardiac catheterization, 35–36
Cardiac diagnostic study, 19–38
Cardiac disorder, 89–103
  aortic, 89–91
  atrial myxoma as, 93
  cardiogenic shock and, 217–219
  congestive heart failure as, 94
  hyperlipidemia and, 97–100
  hypertension as, 100–101
  of mitral valve, 91–93
  pericarditis as, 94–95
  postoperative arrhythmia and, 95
  surgery for, 96–97
Cardiac enzyme, 30
Cardiac isoenzyme, 181
Cardiac magnetic resonance imaging, 33
Cardiac marker, 28–29
Cardiac-specific troponin, 30
Cardiac support device, 199–213
Cardiac tamponade
  trauma causing, 181
  treatment of, 208
Cardiac transplantation, 97
Cardiogenic shock, 217–219
Cardiopulmonary exercise testing, 49
Cardiovascular disorder
  cardiac diagnostic tests in, 22–23
  mechanical ventilation and, 254
  in sepsis, 194
Cardioversion, 209
Carotid artery, 28
Carotid duplex, 15
Carotid stenosis, 15
Catamenial pneumothorax, 85
CD4$^+$ T-cell, HIV infection and, 8, 8t
Cellulitis, 140–141
Centers for Disease Control and Prevention, 161
Central sensitization, 244
Cephalization, 47

Cerebral aneurysm, 116
Cerebral contusion, 188t
Cerebrospinal fluid
  in meningitis, 121t
  in skull fracture, 180
Cervical spinal injury, 185
Chest radiograph
  in cardiac disease, 27
  common views for, 43–44, 45f
  in dyspnea, 14
  in emphysema, 15
  in malignancy, 13
  in pleural effusion, 78
  for pneumothorax, 180t
  in pulmonary embolus, 80
Cholecystitis, 106–107
Cholelithiasis, 106
Cholesterol, 20–21
  coronary artery disease and, 157–158
  levels of, 157t
  serum, 22
Cholestyramine, 100
Christianity, 264
Chronic disease, anemia of, 143t
Chronic gout, 133
Chronic leukemia, 146
Chronic obstructive pulmonary disease, 75–77
Chronic pain, 233
Chronic renal failure, 128
Chylomicron, 21
Cigarette smoking, 76
CK, 29
CK-MB, 29
Classification
  of hemorrhagic shock, 182
  New York Heart Association, 20
Claudication, intermittent, 139–140
Clogging of feeding tube, 174
Clonidine for alcohol withdrawal syndrome, 230
Clostridium difficile, 173–174
Coagulopathy in sepsis, 194
Coccus, 52
Colic, biliary, 106
Colon cancer screening, 159
Colonoscopy, 109
Coma
  hypoglycemia, 65–66
  hypo-osmolar nonketotic, 65
Communication about end-of-life issues, 266–267
Community-acquired pneumonia, 73
Compartment syndrome, 135–136, 186–187
Compensated anemia, 145
Compensatory mechanism in shock, 215–216

Complex partial seizure, 115
Complex regional pain syndrome, 242
Compliance values, 252
Complicated pneumothorax, 84–85
Complications
    of bariatric surgery, 107
    of diabetes, 62
    of diverticulitis, 110
    of enteral feeding, 174
    of mechanical ventilation, 255–256
    of ventricular assist device, 207
    of weaning from ventilator, 256
Compression, spinal cord, 146–147
Computed tomography
    in cardiology, 33–34
    electron beam, 13
    of intra-abdominal injury, 184
    in pulmonary disease, 47–48
    in pulmonary embolus, 80
Congestive heart failure, 94
Consent, informed, 260
Contusion, cerebral, 188t
Conversion, opioid, 239
Coronary arteriography, 35–36
Coronary artery bypass graft, 96–97, 97t
Coronary artery catheterization, 35
Coronary artery disease, 27–28, 35–36
    baseline tests for, 20
    cardiac catheterization in, 36
    lipoprotein and, 157–158
    low-density lipoprotein and, 21
    risk factors for, 19
Corticosteroid
    for anaphylactic shock, 220
    for spinal cord compression, 147
COX II inhibitor, 237
Cranial nerve injury, oculomotor, 179
Creatinine kinase, 29
Crisis, adrenal, 68
CRPS, 242
Cryptococcus meningitis, 121
Crystal, monosodium urate, 133
Culturally sensitive end-of-life care, 262–263
Cushing's disease or syndrome, 67
Cycle, heart, 23–24

D

Dawn phenomenon, 66t
Death
    diabetic ketoacidosis causing, 65
    end-of-life issues and, 259–274
    pneumonia causing, 73–74
    trauma triad of, 183

Débridement of venous stasis ulcer, 139
Debriefing of staff, 270
Decay, tooth, 156
Decision maker, surrogate, 260
Decision making at end of life, 261f
Deep venous thrombosis, 79, 137–138
    bariatric surgery and, 108
    risk factors for, 186t
    trauma and, 185
Delirium, 223–225
Delirium tremens, 230
Demerol, 238
Dental health, 156
Dependence, 243
Deviation, left axis, 24
DEXA scan, 13
    in osteoporosis, 135
DI, 68–69
Diabetes
    prevention of, 156
    types of, 57–58, 57t, 58t, 59t
Diabetes Control and Complications Trial, 67
Diabetes insipidus, 68–69
Diabetic ketoacidosis, 5, 64
    mortality rate for, 65
Diagnostic study
    cardiac, 19–38
    pulmonary, 39–53
    radiological, 13–17
    for seizures, 116
Diaphragm, in chest radiograph, 45
Diarrhea, enteral feedings and, 173–174
Diastolic blood pressure, 100
Diazepam, 225–226
Diffuse axonal injury, 188t
Diffusing capacity of carbon monoxide, 39, 42
Digoxin, 94
Dissection, aortic, 90–91
    magnetic resonance imaging in, 15
Diuretic in congestive heart failure, 94
Diverticulitis, 110, 110t
Diverticulosis, 110
D_LCO, 39, 42
Do not resuscitate order, 267
Donation, organ, 265–266
Doppler echocardiography, 31
Drotrecogin alpha, 196
Drug
    adjuvant, 237
    for diabetes, 60–61, 61t–62t
    for hyperlipidemia, 97–100
    intracerebral hemorrhage caused by, 117

Drug—*cont'd*
  for neuropathic path, 241
  for sedation, 225–226
Dual energy x-ray absorptiometry, 13, 135
Duodenal ulcer, perforated, 105
Durable power of attorney, 259
Dysmetabolic syndrome, 66
Dyspnea, 14

E

ECG, 23–27
Echocardiography
  in cardiac injury, 181
  diagnostic, 30–31
  transesophageal
    advantages of, 15
    in cardiac disease, 31
  transthoracic, in valvular disease, 15
  ventricular assist device and, 205
Economic issues in end of life care, 264
Ectopic activity, ventricular, 34
EECP, 97
Effusion, pleural, 47
  on chest radiograph, 78
Elderly
  fall injury to, 190
  injury prevention for, 162–163
Electrical conduction of heart, 23
Electrocardiography, 23–27, 26f
  in pericarditis, 95
  in pneumothorax, 84
Electrolyte disorder, 3
Electron beam computed tomography, 13, 34
Electrophysiologist, 27
Embolus, pulmonary, 16, 79–80
Emergency
  cellulitis as, 140–141
  intracranial bleeding as, 118
Emphysema, 15, 75–77
Encephalitis, 121–122
End-of-life issues, 259–274, 270f
Endocrine disorder, 55–72
  Cushing's syndrome as, 67–68
    diabetes, 55–67
    diabetes insipidus as, 68–69
    hyperparathyroid, 70
    thyroid, 69–70
Endoscopic retrograde cholangiopancreatography,
  14
Endoscopy, 15
Energy expenditure, 171
Energy requirement, 170
Enhanced external counter pulsation, 97

Enteral therapy, 172–173
  at home, 175
Enzyme, cardiac, 30, 181
Epidural hematoma, 187t
Epigastric pain, 105
Epinephrine for anaphylactic shock, 220
Equianalgesia, opioid, 240t
Escherichia coli causing pyelonephritis, 126–127
Esophagogastroduodenoscopy, 109
Ethics committee, 269
European Society of Cardiology, 28
Euthanasia, 262
Evidence-based treatment for hyperlipidemia, 97
Excretion, of sodium, 6
Exercise stress test, in cardiology, 34
Exercise testing, cardiopulmonary, 49–50
Expiratory pressure, maximum, 43
Expiratory volume, forced, 41
External counter pulsation, enhanced, 97
Extrarenal sodium loss, 4
Extrinsic restrictive lung disease, 40
Extubation, video barium swallow after, 13
Eye examination, 156

F

Fall injury, 190
FAST examination, 184
Fasting glucose, 58
Fever, neutropenic, 149t–150t
Fibric acid, 100
Fibrillation, atrial, postoperative, 93, 95
Five Wishes living will, 271
Fixed mode ventricular assist device, 202
Flolan, 82
Fluid
  cerebrospinal
    in meningitis, 121t
    in skull fracture, 180
    in diabetic ketoacidosis, 64
Fluid resuscitation, 185
Focused assessment by sonography, 184
Folic acid deficiency, 144t
Forced expiratory volume
  in chronic obstructive pulmonary disease, 77
  in obstructive and restrictive disease, 41
Forced vital capacity, 41
Formula
  for corrected calcium, 7
  enteral, 172–173
  Parkland, 185
Fractional excretion of sodium, 6
Fracture
  compartment syndrome and, 186

Fracture—*cont'd*
pelvic, 181–182
FT$_4$I, 10
Fungal meningitis, 121
FVC, 41

G

Gap, anion, 5
Gastric emptying, 173
Gastrointestinal bleeding, 15, 108–110
Gastrointestinal disorder, 105–113
barietric surgery and, 107–108
biliary colic as, 106–107
diverticular, 110–111
enteral feedings and, 173
obstruction as, 107, 111–112
pain in, 105
pancreatitis as, 106
perforated duodenal ulcer as, 105
in sepsis, 195
Gemfibrozil, 100
Generalized seizure, 115
Genitourinary disorder, 125–130
GI bleed, 108–110
Glaucoma screening, 155–156
Glomerulonephritis, 129
Glucose
fasting, 58
in total parenteral nutrition, 172
Glucose tolerance, 58
Glycosylated hemoglobin, 60
Gout, 133–134
Grading system for cardiac biopsy, 37t
Graft, coronary artery bypass, 96–97
Gram-negative bacteria, 52
Gram-positive bacteria, 52
Gram stain, sputum, 51
Guardianship, 259
Guidelines, American College of Cardiology/
American Heart Association, 27
Gum disease, 156

H

Haemophilus influenzae, 73
Haemophilus influenzae vaccine, 184
Haloperidol for delirium, 226
Hashimoto's thyroiditis, 70
HbA1c, 60
HbsAB, 9
HbsAG, 9
Health promotion, 155–164
Healthy People 2010, 155

Heart
cardiogenic shock and, 217–219
in chest radiograph, 44
diagnostic tests of, 19–38
electrical conduction of, 23
electron beam computed tomography of, 13
Heart cycle, 23–24
Heart failure, congestive, 94
Heart transplantation, 94, 97
Heart valve abnormality, 15
Hematological disorder, 143–152
anemia as, 143–144
leukemia as, 144
neutropenic, 148–150
in sepsis, 194
thrombocytopenia as, 150–151
Hematologist, referral to, 7
Hematoma
liver, 189
subdural, 187t
Hematuria, 125
Hemodynamics
in cardiogenic shock and, 217–218
in sepsis, 194
Hemoglobin, glycosylated, 60
Hemorrhage
gastrointestinal, 15, 108–110
intracerebral, 117–118
subarachnoid, 118, 188t
Hemorrhagic shock
classification, 182t
hypotension in, 182
Hemorrhagic stroke, 116
Hemothorax, 180t
Heparin-induced thrombocytopenia, 150–151,
150t–151t, 210
Hepatic disorder in sepsis, 195
Hepatitis A virus, 9
Hepatitis B vaccine, 163
Hepatitis C virus, 9
Hepatobiliary scan, 13
Herpes simplex virus encephalitis, 122
HIDA scan, 13–14
High-density lipoprotein, 21
Hila, 44
Hinduism, 264
History, patient, of stroke, 119
HIV infection, 8, 8t, 161
Holter monitor, 26
Home care
nutritional therapy and, 175
ventricular assist device and, 211

Homocysteine, 22
Honeycombing, 47
Hormone. *See* Endocrine disorder
Hospice, 268–269
Hospital-acquired pneumonia, 74–75
Human immunodeficiency virus infection, 161
   CD4+ T-cells and, 8, 8t
Human leukocyte antigen, 8
Hydration with enteral therapy, 172–173
Hypercapnia, 248–249
Hypercoagulation, 6
Hyperkalemia, 5
   in diabetic ketoacidosis, 64
Hyperlipidemia, 97–100, 98f–100t
Hyperparathyroidism, 70
Hypersensitivity reaction, 219–220
Hypertension, 100–101
   aortic dissection and, 91
   intra-abdominal, 184
Hypertonic hyponatremia, 4
Hypoglycemic agent, 60–61
Hypoglycemic coma, 65–66
Hyponatremia, 3–4
   in diabetic ketoacidosis, 64
   syndrome of inappropriate secretion of
      antidiuretic hormone and, 5
Hypoparathyroidism, 70
Hyposomolar nonketotic syndrome, 65
Hypotension in hemorrhagic shock, 182
Hypovolemic shock, 216–217
Hypoxia, 248

I

I-time, 249
ICH, 117–118
ICU psychosis, 230
I:E ratio, 252, 254
Iloprost, 83
Immune-mediated thrombocytopenia, 150–151
Immunization
   influenza, 161
   tetanus, 190
Implantation of ventricular assist device,
   199–200
IMT, 28
Incapacitated person, 259–260
Incompetent patient, 260–261
Index
   ankle-brachial blood pressure, 27–28
   body mass, 169–170, 170t
Index of Rapid and Shallow Breathing, 256
Infarction, myocardial, 28

Infection
   cellulitis, 140–141
   common sites of, 196
   hepatitis A, 9
   hepatitis C, 9
   HIV, CD4+ cell count in, 8
   meningitis, 120–121
   necrotizing, 141
   pneumonia, 73–75
   pyelonephritis, 126–127
   risk factors for, 7
   tube feeding and, 174
   tuberculosis, 77–78
Infection prophylaxis with cardiac assist device,
   208–209
Infiltrate, pulmonary, 46
Inflammation
   diverticular, 110
   pericardial, 94–95
Inflammatory response syndrome, systemic,
   193–194
Influenza immunization, 161
Informed consent, 260
Injury, traumatic, 179–191
   prevention of, in elderly, 162–163
Inspiratory pressure, maximum, 43
Inspiratory time, 249
Insulin, types of, 63, 63t
Insulin resistance syndrome, 66
Insulin secretogogue, 60
Insulin sensitizer, 61, 62t
Insurance for nutritional services, 175–176
Intensive care unit, psychosis in, 230
Intermittent claudication, 139–140
Internet resources
   for cardiac disease, 38
   for cardiac disorders, 102
   for diagnostic studies, 11
   for end-of-life issues, 272
   for endocrine disorders, 71
   for health promotion, 163
   for hematological disorder, 152
   on mechanical ventilation, 257
   on musculoskeletal and vascular disorders, 142
   on neurological disorder, 122
   for nutrition, 175–176
   for pain management, 244
   for pulmonary disease, 53, 87
   on renal and gGenitourinary disorders, 130
   for sedation, 231
   on sepsis, 197
   for shock, 220

Internet resources—*cont'd*
    on trauma, 190
        for ventricular assist device and, 213
Interstitial nephritis, 129
Interstitial pulmonary infiltrate, 46
Intimal medial thickness of carotid artery, 28
Intra-abdominal hypertension, 184
Intra-abdominal injury, 184
Intraaortic balloon pump, 218
Intracerebral hemorrhage, 117–118
Intracompartmental pressure, 135–136
Intracorporeal ventricular assist device, 205
Intracranial bleeding, 118
Intravenous pyelogram, 14
Intrinsic restrictive lung disease, 40
Intubation, video barium swallow after, 13
Inverse I:E ratio, 252
Iron-binding capacity, 7–8
Iron-deficiency anemia, 143
    testing for, 7
Islam, 264
Isoform, 29
Isotonic hyponatremia, 4
IV adenosine in stress testing, 35

J
Jaundice, 14
Joint, gout and, 133–134
Joint Commission on Accreditation of Healthcare
    Organizations, 233
Judaism, 264

K
Kappa receptor, 235, 235t
Kerley B lines, 47
Kernig sign, 121
Ketoacidosis, diabetic, 5

L
Laceration, liver, 189
Lactic dehydrogenase, 29–30
Laparotomy, 189
Large bowel obstruction, 107, 111t–112t
Lateral chest radiograph, 43
Lateral decubitus chest radiograph, 44
Lavage, peritoneal, 182
LDH, 29–30
Leak, anastomotic, 107
Left axis deviation, 24
Left ventricular assist device, 206f, 209
Left ventricular dysfunction, 34
Leukemia, 144

Leukocyte esterase, 10
Life support, withdrawing of, 271
Lipid, 20–21
Lipoprotein, 20–21
    coronary artery disease and, 157–158
    types of, 22
Liver
    injury to, 189, 189t
    sepsis and, 195
Liver function, blood testing for, 6
Living will, 260
Lordotic chest radiograph, 44
Lovastatin, 99
Low-density lipoprotein, 21
    coronary artery disease and, 157–158
    diabetes and, 62
Lower quadrant pain, 105
Lumbar spinal injury, 185
Lung cancer, 160
Lung capacity, 39
    in obstructive and restrictive disease, 41
Lung fields, 45
Lung volume, 39
Lymphoblastic leukemia, 145, 146

M
Macrovascular complications of diabetes, 62
Magnetic resonance angiography in renal artery
    stenosis, 14
Magnetic resonance imaging
    in aortic dissection, 15
    in cardiology, 33
    in pulmonary disease, 48
    of St. Jude mechanical valve, 15
    for spinal cord compression, 146
Malformation, vascular, 116–117
Malignancy
    chest x-ray in, 13
    pain in, 238
    screening for, 158–160
    spinal cord compression and, 146–147
    thyroid, 69–70
Malignant pericardial disease, 148
Malnutrition, 167, 169
Marker
    cardiac, 28–29
    for hepatitis A, 9
Maximal voluntary ventilation, 42–43
Maximum expiratory pressure, 43
Maximum inspiratory pressure, 43
Meatus, urethral, blood in, 182
Mechanical valve, St. Jude, 15

Mechanical ventilation, 247–258
  indications for, 249
  microorganisms and, 75
Medial thickness, intimal, 28
Mediastinum, 44
Medicare, end of life and, 264
Meglitinide, 60–61, 62t
Meningitis, 120–121, 121t
Meningitis vaccination, 162
  after splenectomy, 184
MET, 34
Metabolic acidosis, 51
Metabolic alkalosis, 51
Metabolic equivalent, 34
Microvascular complications of diabetes,
  62–63
Midazolam, 225
Mild pain, 237
Mind-body therapy for pain, 243
Minute ventilation, 251
Mitral valve prolapse, 91
Mitral valvular regurgitation, 92
Mnemonic, VINDICATE, 236, 237t
MODS, 194
Monitor, Holter, 26–27
Monitoring
  of parenteral or enteral feeding, 175
  of sedation therapy, 226–227
  of ventilator, 250–251
Monosodium urate crystal, 133
Morphine, 238
Mortality
  diabetic ketoacidosis and, 65
  end-of-life issues and, 259–274
  pneumonia and, 73–74
Motor activity assessment scale, 229, 229t
MRA, 14
MRI. See Magnetic resonance imaging
Mu receptor, 235, 235t
MUGA scan, 32
Multidisciplinary approach to pain management,
  243–244
Multigated acquisition scan, 32
Multiple organ dysfunction syndrome, 194
Muscles of respiration, 73
Musculoskeletal disorder, 133–137
Mycobacterium tuberculosis, 77–78
Myelogenous leukemia, 145, 146
Myocardial dysfunction in cardiogenic shock,
  218
Myocardial infarction, 28
Myocardial ischemia, 34

Myocardial revascularization, 96
Myoglobin, 30
Myxoma, atrial, 93

N
National Guidelines Clearinghouse, 97
Natriuretic peptide, B-type, 22
Neck injury, 187
Necrotizing infection, 141
Nephritis, interstitial, 129
Nephrolithiasis, 125–126
Nephropathy, diabetic, 63
Neurogenic shock, 220–221
Neurological disorder, 115–123
  brain tumor as, 119–120
  cerebral aneurysm as, 116
  hemorrhagic stroke as, 116
  intracerebral hemorrhage as, 117–118
  meningitis as, 120–121
  seizure as, 115–116
  in sepsis, 195
  stroke as, 118–119
  subarachnoid hemorrhage as, 118
  vascular malformation as, 116–117
Neuromuscular restrictive lung disease, 40
Neuropathic pain, 236, 241–242
Neuropathy, diabetic, 63
Neurotransmitter, pain, 235t
Neutropenic disorder, 148–149, 149t–150t
Neutrophil count, 7
New York Heart Association classification, 20
Niacin, 100
Nicotinic acid, 100
Nitrite in urine, 10
Nodule
  pulmonary, 47
  solitary, 75
  thyroid, 69–70
Nonpenetrating trauma
  aortic, 180–181
  cardiac, 181
  pneumothorax and, 85
Nonsteroidal antiinflammatory drug
  for gout, 134
  in pericarditis, 95
Norepinephrine for sepsis, 196
Normal sinus rhythm, 24–25
Northwest axis, 24
Nosocomial pneumonia, 74
Nuclear cardiology, 31
Nutrition, 167–176
  admission assessment of, 168t–169t

Nutrition—*cont'd*
    mass body index and, 170t
Nutritional supplementation, 171

O

Obesity, 160
    body mass index and, 170
Oblique chest radiograph, 43
Obstruction
    airway, reversible, 42
    bowel, 107, 111t–112t
Obstructive jaundice, 14
Obstructive lung disease, 40
Obstructive pulmonary disease, chronic, 75–77
Occult blood, 159
Occult pneumothorax, 180t
Off-pump coronary artery bypass graft, 96
Oncological disorder
    leukemia as, 144
    pericardial, 148
    spinal cord compression as, 146–147
    superior vena cava syndrome as, 147–148
Opioid
    long-acting, 238
    for sedation, 225
    side effects of, 240
    withdrawal from, 240–241
Opioid equianalgesia, 240t
Oral hypoglycemic agent, 60–61, 61t–62t
Order, do not resuscitate, 267
Organ donation, 265–266
Organ system dysfunction in sepsis, 194–195
Osmolality, 3
Osteoarthritis, 134
Osteoporosis, 134–135
    risk factors for, 156–157
Oxycodone, 238
Oxygen consumption, 50
Oxygen therapy, 50
Oxygenation, 250

P

P wave, 25
PaCO$_2$, 250
Pain, 233–246
    abdominal, 105
    acute versus chronic, 233
    assessment of, 236
    breakthrough, 237
    cancer, 238
    complex regional, 242
    endogenous opioids and, 235
    epigastric, 105

    of gout, 133
    of intermittent claudication, 139
    mind-body therapy for, 243
    multidisciplinary approach to, 243–244
    neuropathic, 236, 241–242
    opioids for, 238–241
    somatic, 236
    transmission of, 233–235, 234f, 235t
    of venous stasis ulcer, 139
    visceral, 236
Palliative care, 268–269
Palliative terminal care, 262
Pancreatitis, 106
Papanicolaou test, 158, 160
Paracorporeal ventricular assist device, 205
Parenteral nutrition, 171–172
    at home, 175
Parkland formula, 185
Partial pressure of arterial carbon dioxide, 250
Partial seizure, 115
Patient-controlled analgesia, 238–239
Patient Self-Determination Act, 262
Peak pressures, 249
Pelvic examination, 160
Pelvic fracture, 181–182
Penetrating trauma
    pneumothorax caused by, 85
    to small bowel, 189
Peptide, B-type natriuretic, 22
Perforation
    diverticular, 110
    of duodenal ulcer, 105
Perfusion, low, 251
Perfusion imaging, 32
Pericardial disease, malignant, 148
Pericarditis, 94–95
Peripheral parenteral nutrition, 171
Peritoneal lavage, 182
PET scan, 33
Pharmacologic stress testing, 35
Pharmacological agent. *See* Drug
Phlebitis, superficial, 138
Physical dependence, 243
Pink puffer, 76
Plaque in coronary artery disease, 21
Plateau pressure, 251
Pleura, 45
Pleural effusion, 47
    on chest radiograph, 78
Pneumonia
    atypical, 75
    community-acquired, 73
    mortality rate for, 73–74

Pneumonia—*cont'd*
  ventilator-associated, 255–256
Pneumothorax, 47, 83
  chest radiograph for, 180t
  primary, 83
  secondary, 84–85
Pneumovax after splenectomy, 184
Positive end-expiratory pressure, 249
Positron emission tomography
  in cardiology, 33
  pulmonary, 49
Posteroanterior chest radiograph, 43, 44, 445f
Postmenopausal bone loss, 157
Postpartum thyroiditis, 70
Postvoid residual, 14
Potassium
  in diabetic ketoacidosis, 64
  hyperkalemia and, 5
  T waves and, 23
Power of attorney, 259
PQRST complex, 23
PR interval, 25
Precautions, neutropenic, 148–149
Pressure
  intracompartmental, 135–136
  maximum expiratory, 43
  maximum inspiratory, 43
  plateau, 251
Pressure ventilation, 249
Prevention
  of anaphylactic shock, 220
  of aspiration, 173
  of breast cancer, 157
  of coronary artery disease, 158
  of nosocomial pneumonia, 74–75
  of osteoporosis, 156–157
  of sepsis, 196–197
Prolapse, mitral valve, 91
Prophylaxis
  with cardiac assist device, 208–209
  tetanus, 190
Propofol, 226
Prostacyclin, 82
Prostate-specific antigen, 9, 158
Protein
  C-reactive, 22
  requirement for, 171
  in urine, 10
Protein-energy malnutrition, 167
Protein status, visceral, 170, 170t
Pseudoaddiction, 243
Pseudohyponatremia, 4
Psychological dependence, 243

Psychosis, ICU, 230
Pulmonary angiography, 16
Pulmonary diagnostic study, 39–53
Pulmonary disorder
  asthma as, 85–86
  chronic obstructive, 75–77
  pleural effusion as, 78–79
  plmonary hypertension as, 80–82
  pneumonia as, 73–75
  pneumothorax as, 83–85
  pulmonary embolus as, 16, 79–80
  pulmonary nodule as, 75
  tuberculosis as, 77–78
Pulmonary embolus, 79–80
  angiography in, 16
Pulmonary function test, 39
  in obstructive and restrictive disease, 40–41
Pulmonary hypertension, 80–82
Pulmonary infiltrate, 46
Pulmonary nodule, 47, 75
Pulse-dose steroid for chronic obstructive
  pulmonary disease, 77
Pump
  intraaortic balloon, 218
  ventricular assist, 200
Pupil, blown, 179
Pyelogram, intravenous, 14
Pyelonephritis, 126–127

Q
QRS axis, 25
QRS complex, normal, 25
QRS segment, 23
QT interval, 25

R
Radiation therapy for spinal cord compression,
  147
Radiography
  diagnostic, 13–17
  in spinal injury, 188
Radioisotope in cardiology, 31–32
Ramsay scale, 227, 227t
RAS, 14
Ratio
  BUN/creatinine, 10
  V/Q, 16
Receptor, analgesic, 235, 235t
Refeeding syndrome, 174–175
Referral to hematologist, 7
Regional pain syndrome, complex, 242
Regurgitation, mitral vavular, 92
Relaxation phase of heart cycle, 23

Religion, 263–264
Remodulin, 83
Renal artery stenosis, 14
Renal disorder, 125–130
   in sepsis, 194
Renal failure, 128–129, 128t
Renal sodium loss, 4
Residual, postvoid, 14
Resources
   end-of-life care and, 264, 271
   Internet. *See* Internet resources
   on ventricular assist device, 211
Respiration, muscles of, 73
Respiratory alkalosis, 51
Respiratory disorder in sepsis, 194
Respiratory failure, 247t–248t
Respiratory values, 249–250
Restrictive lung disease, 40
Resuscitation
   fluid, 185
   of terminally ill patient, 268
Retention, urinary, 14, 127
Reticulocyte count, 7
Retrograde urethrogram, 182
Revascularization, myocardial, 96
Reversible airway obstruction, 42
Rheumatoid arthritis, 133–134
Rhythm, sinus, 24–25
Rib in chest radiograph, 45
Richmond agitation-sedation scale, 227,
   227t–228t
Right-to-die amendment, 262
Right ventricular assist device, 206f
Right ventricular dysfunction, 208
Riker sedation-agitation scale, 228–229, 228t
Risk factors
   for coronary artery disease, 19
   for deep venous thrombosis, 186
   for infection, 7
   for malnutrition, 167
   for osteoporosis, 156–157
   for sepsis, 193

S

St. Jude mechanical valve, 15
Salt, limiting of, 158
Sao₂, 251
Scale, angiation-sedation, 227–228
Scan
   DEXA, 13
   multigated acquisition, 32
Scintillation, in cardiology, 31–32
Score, cardiac calcium, 13

Screening
   cancer, 158–160
   diabetes, 58
   glaucoma, 155–156
   for hypercoagulation, 6
   nutrition risk, 167–169
   as prevention, 155
Secretogogue, insulin, 60
Sedation management, 223–232, 224t, 227t, 228t,
   229t
Seizure, 115–116, 115t
Sensitization, central, 244
Sepsis, risk factors for, 193
Septic shock, 194, 195
Serological marker for hepatitis A, 9
Serum cardiac marker, 28–29
Serum cholesterol, 22
Serum ferritin, 7
Serum osmolality, 3
Sexually active woman, 160
Shock, 215–222
   anaphylactic, 219–220
   cardiogenic, 217–219
   compensatory mechanism for, 215–216
   definition of, 215
   hemorrhagic
      classification of, 182t
      hypotension in, 182
   hypovolemic, 216–217
   neurogenic, 220–221
   septic, 194, 195
   treatment goals for, 216
SHOCK trial, 218–219
Sickle cell anemia, 144t
Side effects, opioid, 240
Sigma receptor, 235, 235t
Sign
   Brudzinski, 121
   Kernig, 121
   silhouette, 47
Signal-averaged ECG, 26
Silhouette sign, 47
Simple partial seizure, 115
Simple pneumothorax, 83
Sinus rhythm, 24–25
Six-minute walk test, 50
Skin, cellulitis of, 140–141
Skull fracture, 180
Small bowel
   obstruction of, 107, 111t–112t
   penetrating trauma to, 189
Smoking, chronic obstructive pulmonary disease
   and, 76

Sodium
   in diabetic ketoacidosis, 64
   fractional excretion of, 6
   hyponatremia and, 3
   renal and extrarenal losses of, 4
Soft tissue in chest radiograph, 45
Solitary pulmonary nodule, 75
Somatic pain, 236
Somogyi effect, 66t
Sonography in trauma, 184
SPECT test, cardiac, 33
Spinal cord compression, 146–147
Spinal cord injury, 180
Spirometry, 39
Splenectomy, vaccinations after, 184
Spontaneous pneumothorax, 84–85
Sputum Gram stain, 51
ST segment, 23, 25
Staphylococcus aureus pneumonia, 73
Stasis ulcer, venous, 138–139
Static compliance, 252
Statin, 99
Stenosis
   aortic, 89–90
   carotid, 15
   renal artery, 14
Sternum, 45
Steroid
   for chronic obstructive pulmonary disease, 77
   in sepsis, 196
Stool in bowel obstruction, 111
Streptococcus pneumoniae, 73
Stress echocardiography, 35
Stress test, exercise, 34
Stricture, intestinal, 107, 108
Stroke, 118–119
   hemorrhagic, 116
Study to Understand Prognoses and Preferences
   for Outcomes and Risks of Treatment, 263
Subacute thyroiditis, 70
Subarachnoid hemorrhage, 118, 187, 188t
Subcutaneous tissue, cellulitis of, 140–141
Subdural hematoma, 187t
Sulfonylurea, 60
Sulfur colloid scan, for bleeding, 109
Sun protection factor, 160
Superficial phlebitis, 138
Superior vena cava syndrome, 147–148
SUPPORT trial, 263
Surgery
   bariatric, 107–108
   cardiac valve replacement, 90
   for mitral vavular regurgitation, 92

for pneumothorax, 84
   in trauma, 183t
Surrogate decision maker, 260
Swallow, barium, video, 13
Syndrome of inappropriate secretion of
   antidiuretic hormone, 5
Syndrome X, 66
Systemic inflammatory response syndrome,
   193–194
Systolic blood pressure, 100

T
T lymphocyte, CD4$^+$, 8
T wave, 23, 25–26
Tagged red blood cell scan, 109
Tamponade
   trauma causing, 181
   treatment of, 208
TEE, 31
Tension pneumothorax, 85, 180, 180t
Terminally ill patient, 259–274
Tetanus prophylaxis, 190
Thallium stress test, 35
Theophylline, 77
Thiazolidinedione, 61
Thoracentesis, 79
Thoracic spinal injury, 185
Thoratec Heartmate, 201, 202f
Thoratec paracorporeal device, 200, 202f
3 in 1 rule, 185
Thrombocytopenia, heparin-induced, 150–151,
   150t–151t, 210
Thrombolytic therapy, 80
Thrombosis, deep venous, 79, 137–138
   bariatric surgery and, 108
   risk factors for, 186t
   trauma and, 185
Thyroid disease, FT$_4$I in, 10
Thyroid disorder, 69–70
Thyroiditis, 70
Tidal volume, 249
Tolerance, 243
Tooth decay, 156
Total iron-binding capacity, 7–8
Total lung capacity, 41
Total parenteral nutrition, 171–172
   at home, 175
Tracleer, 82
Tramadol, 240
Transesophageal echocardiography, 15, 31
Transmyocardial revascularization, 97
Transplantation
   cardiac, 94

Transplantation—*cont'd*
  donation for, 265–266
  heart, 97
Transthoracic echocardiography
  in cardiac injury, 181
  in valvular disease, 15
Trauma, 179–191
  pneumothorax caused by, 85
Trauma triad of death, 183
Travel, ventricular assist device and, 211
Triad
  Beck's, 181
  of death, 183
Triglyceride, 21
Tube feeding, 172–175
Tuberculosis, 77–78, 161
Tumor, brain, 119–120
Twelve-lead electrocardiography, 24–25
Typical angina pectoris, 19

U

U wave, 26, 26f
Ulcer
  duodenal, perforated, 105
  venous stasis, 138–139
Ultram, 240
Ultrasonography, in urinary retention, 14
Ultraviolet wave, 160
Uncompensated anemia, 145
United Kingdom Prospective Diabetes Study, 67
United States Preventive Services Task Force, 155,
  162
Upper gastrointestinal bleeding, 15
Upper quadrant pain, 105
Urethral meatus, blood in, 182
Uric acid, 133
Urinalysis in renal failure, 128, 128t
Urinary retention, 14, 127
Urine
  blood in, 125
  nitrites in, 10
  protein in, 10

V

V/Q mismatch, 251
V/Q ratio, 16
V/Q scan, 48
  in pulmonary embolus, 16, 80
Vaccination, 162
  after splenectomy, 184
  meningitis, 162
Vaccine, tetanus, 190
VAD, 199–213

Valve, cardiac, 89–93
  aortic, 89–91
  mitral, 91–93
  St. Jude, 15
  transthoracic echocardiography of, 15
Valve replacement surgery, 90
Vascular complications of diabetes, 62–63
Vascular disorder, 137–140
  coronary artery, 19, 20
  pulmonary hypertension as, 80–82
Vascular injury, 182–183
Vascular malformation, 116–117
Vascular study in coronary artery disease, 27
Vasoconstrictor in anaphylaxis, 220
Vasopressin in sepsis, 196
Ve, 251
Vena cava syndrome, superior, 147–148
Venous stasis ulcer, 138–139
Venous thrombosis, deep, 79, 137–138
  bariatric surgery and, 108
  risk factors for, 186t
  trauma and, 185
Venous versus arterial injury, 182–183
Ventilation
  maximal voluntary, 42–43
  mechanical, 75
Ventilation/perfusion scan, 48
  in pulmonary embolus, 16, 80
Ventilator alarm, 254–255
Ventilator-associated pneumonia, 255–256
Ventilator management, 247–258
Ventilator mode, 252, 252t–253t
Ventricular assist device, 199–213
Ventricular dysfunction
  left, 34
  right, 208
Ventricular ectopic activity, 34
Vertebra in chest radiograph, 45
Very low density lipoprotein, 21
Vest scan, 32
Video barium swallow, 13
VINDICATE mnemonic, 236, 237t
Viral encephalitis, 121–122
Viral infection
  hepatitis, 9
  prevention of, 161
Viral load in HIV infection, 8
Visceral pain, 236
Visceral protein status, 170, 170t
Vital capacity, forced, 41
Vitamin B_{12} deficiency, 144t
VO_2, 50
Volume ventilation, 249

Voluntary ventilation, maximal, 42–43
Vomiting in bowel obstruction, 111

W
Walk test, 6-minute, 50
Wave, ultraviolet, 160
Weaning from ventilator, 256
Withdrawal, opioid, 240–241
Withholding of life support, 271

World Health Organization, on cancer pain, 238
World Heart Novacor, 202, 202f

X
Xigris therapy, 196

Z
Zones of injury in neck, 187

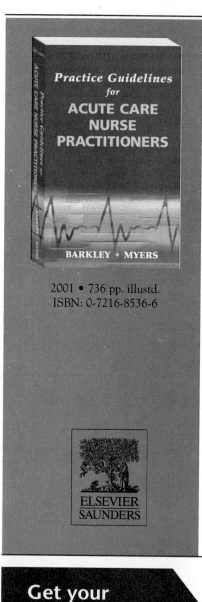